The Psychiatry of Palliative Medicine

The dying mind

Dr A D (Sandy) Macleod
MBChB, FRANZCP, FAChPM
Consultant Psychiatrist, Christchurch Hospital
and Medical Director, Nurse Maude Hospice,
Christchurch, New Zealand

Foreword by

Ian Maddocks

Radcliffe Publishing
Oxford ● New York

Radcliffe Publishing Ltd
18 Marcham Road
Abingdon
Oxon OX14 1AA
United Kingdom

www.radcliffe-oxford.com
Electronic catalogue and worldwide online ordering facility.

British Library Cataloguing in Publication Data

A catalogue record for this book is available from the British Library.

ISBN-10: 1 84619 092 4
ISBN-13: 978 1 84619 092 6

Typeset by Aarontype Ltd, Easton, Bristol, UK
Printed and bound by Biddles Ltd, King's Lynn, Norfolk, UK

Contents

Foreword

Palliative medicine began with quite a narrow focus on the management of the terminal phase of advanced cancer. During the last decade, however, its relevance to other specialties has been increasingly recognised, finding expression in articles and monographs relating to the advanced stages of cardiac, respiratory and neurological diseases. It may be considered strange that psychiatry has not received similar prominence, since psychiatry has always been a potential partner of palliative medicine. Illness that threatens imminent death challenges the mental and social well-being of affected individuals and their families. Consistent specialist psychiatric care has nevertheless not been readily available to the dying. In some communities this may be due to a shortage of trained psychiatrists. Also relevant, however, has been the drive to have palliative medicine recognised as a specialty of internal medicine, encouraging an emphasis on symptom management, drug therapies and evidence-based practice, with the risk of a lesser status for behavioural aspects of care.

Because there may never be sufficient numbers of psychiatrists interested in bringing their expertise to this field, working with the dying mind depends on staff with limited training in behavioural medicine and psychiatry. To redress the inadequate engagement of psychiatry, Sandy Macleod has concentrated on those important areas in palliative medicine where a pragmatic knowledge of psychiatry can make a difference. Here is sensible guidance that will enable staff to serve their client patients and families more adequately.

Short didactic sentences offer commendable clarity; and some will, I hope, become favourite aphorisms for the discipline: 'physical examination of the terminally ill is predominantly a psychological exercise'; 'psychologically healthy persons do their own psychotherapy' and 'the nurse is a powerful analgesic'.

The apt quotes that introduce each chapter place the discussion in a long historical context. They remind readers that humans have experienced the discomforts of dying through many millennia. The basic rules of management that medical writers of antiquity proposed remain applicable today. Commonsense assessment ('be careful about making normality into pathology') and simple techniques of touch and building relationship ('chats under the shower') are allowed to sit easily alongside the techniques and pharmacopoeia of modern psychiatry.

An accessible vocabulary free from jargon is important. Palliative care staff will be glad to prefer 'distress' to 'adjustment disorder'. Useful messages for staff well-being include the consequences of being idealised by their patients, and that burn-out has more to do with management and team hygiene than daily contact with dying persons.

We who practice palliative medicine rarely can restore to our patients the comfort, dignity and function to which they aspire. Do they lose hope?

Embedded in Macleod's term 'covenant of acceptance' is the offer of a realistic hope, one in which staff, family and patient may all conspire. I find this an immensely sympathetic book, beautifully written. It is a testimony to the summation of specialist psychiatric knowledge, broad scholarship and a rich personal practice in bedside palliation.

Ian Maddocks
Emeritus Professor of Palliative Care
Flinders University of South Australia
January 2007

Preface

This is a book for clinicians, written by a clinician practising both psychiatry and palliative medicine. Hopefully, it may better inform medical and nursing practitioners about the psychiatry of relevance to the terminally ill. It is a distillation of clinical knowledge, observation and experience, the current medical literature (evidence-based where available) and the opinions and biases of the author. Brevity necessitates incomplete consideration of all aspects of the subject. I have therefore concentrated upon those clinical predicaments that frequently demand a pragmatic knowledge of psychiatry. It will not be appreciated by all; however highlighted are some clinical issues and concepts of management that to date have been rather ignored by palliative medicine.

Sandy Macleod
January 2007
(ad.macleod@cdhb.govt.nz)

About the author

Dr Sandy Macleod graduated from the University of Otago in 1974. After several years of locuming in general practice in New Zealand and the UK Dr Macleod completed his specialist training in psychiatry in Dunedin, New Zealand. Periods of study in Oklahoma City, Boston and London followed.

Since 1985 Dr Macleod has worked as a consultation–liaison psychiatrist/neuropsychiatrist at Christchurch and Burwood Hospitals, Christchurch, New Zealand. In 1993 during tenure as visiting psychiatrist to Burwood Hospice, the illness of the medical officer and the persuasion of the nursing staff enticed Dr Macleod to commence an additional career in palliative care. Juggling busy clinical practices in neuropsychiatry and palliative medicine is demanding and challenging. The pleasures of being able to practise psychiatry within medicine have been immense.

The co-author of a popular regional palliative care handbook, Dr Macleod has also published over fifty articles, chapters and letters about clinical and historical topics in psychiatry and palliative medicine.

Acknowledgements

This book is a tribute to the many thousands of patients whom I have had the privilege to attend in over three decades of medical practice. Many are now sadly deceased. They have taught me a great deal. Of my medical teachers Keith Macleod and Roy Muir deserve special recognition. Tom Hackett, Alwyn Lishman and Ian Maddocks all so willingly, and often from afar, provided me wonderful support and mentoring. My particular thanks to my long-suffering colleagues for their assistance with the various drafts of this manuscript. They include Prabha Chandra, Santosh Chaturvedi, James Lehman, Rod MacLeod, Anne Morgan, Kate Reid and Jane Vella-Brincat.

The author gratefully acknowledges permission to reproduce the following copyright material in this book:

Auden WH. *In Memory of WB Yeats*. © 1940 and renewed 1968 by WH Auden. From *Collected Poems* by WH Auden. Reproduced with permission from Random House and Faber & Faber.

Byrd RE. *Alone: The classic polar adventure*. Reproduced with permission from Island Press.

Gubrich-Simitis I. *Sigmund Freud: his life in pictures and words*. Reproduced with permission from The University of Queensland Press.

Sophocles. Philoctetes. In: D Grene and R Lattimore (eds) *The Complete Greek Tragedies*. Reproduced with permission from The University of Chicago Press.

Stewart, S. *Give Us This Day*. Reproduced with permission from The Balkin Agency.

Strauss MB. *Familiar Medical Quotations*. Reproduced with permission from Lippincott, Williams & Wilkins.

Yeats WB. *The Tower*. Reproduced with permission from Simon & Schuster and AP Watt on behalf of Michael B Yeats.

Every effort has been made to acknowledge correctly and to contact the copyright holders of citations considered in excess of 'fair use'. The author and publishers apologise for any unintentional errors or omissions, which will be corrected in future editions of this book.

Chapter 1

Psychiatry and palliative medicine

It is the special vocation of the doctor to grow familiar with suffering.
John Greenleaf Whittier (1807–1892)[1]

The cardinal goal of medical care is to alleviate suffering. Suffering is an unpleasant and distressing emotional experience that undermines quality of life.[2] When illness confronts the integrity of how we define ourselves, of how we function, of what roles we perform, and how we perceive ourselves, suffering eventuates. The individual's personhood is threatened by an event such as disease.[3] Illness erodes 'the self', and suffering is the symptom of this damage. Suffering encompasses physical, psychological, spiritual and philosophical aspects of the person. Medicine does not have armamentarium to address all the components of suffering induced by disease. Suffering in advanced cancer patients cannot be eliminated, but if adequate relief is achieved then coping and personal growth can occur.[4] Multidisciplinary healthcare teams are necessary to tackle this challenge. Modern medicine, preoccupied by curing rather than caring, focuses on biology rather than psychology and sociology. The fragmentation of medicine, made inevitable by the huge clinical and scientific knowledge base, distracts from the commonalities between the various specialties and subspecialties. Psychiatry and palliative medicine attend patients who are mentally distressed and dying. Neither condition is easily amenable to biomedical interventions. These 'old-fashioned' medical specialties practise biopsychosocial medicine with as much artistry as science. The clinical outcome in psychiatry is 'good' palliation of mental distress. In palliative medicine it is a 'good death'. The diseases of neither patient group are curable. The best that can be achieved is symptom control and maintenance of that control. Quality of (remaining) life is thereby improved and some suffering relieved.

Terminally ill patients can develop psychiatric illness. The provision of specialist psychiatric care to the dying is sporadic and inadequate. Some fortunate patients are seen through consultation–liaison psychiatric services to general hospitals. Psychiatrists rarely venture off their patch and into palliative care facilities. Despite the interest and want of a few psychiatrists, this situation is unlikely to change. Finlay correctly points out the variability of the provision of consultation–liaison services throughout the UK.[5] The decline of consultation–liaison psychiatric services worldwide over the last two decades, because neither mental health nor medical services are willing to fund these services despite their being appreciated and effective, makes the reality of better access to psychiatry unlikely. A 'solution' is that of enhancing the psychiatric skills of palliative care practitioners and fostering the partnership. In the foundation period of modern palliative medicine the deficits identified were those of 'communication skills'. More recently, depression, the psychosocial aspects of pain, and delirium have been areas of educational endeavour. The claiming of palliative medicine by physicians' colleges, and the narrow base of specialist medicine training, have resulted in very limited exposure to psychiatry by prospective palliative medicine specialists. Palliative care nurses usually possess considerable experience and intuitive skill in dealing with disturbed patients, but lack a sound psychiatric knowledge base. As palliative care is slowly expanding outside its traditional oncology base into neurological, cardiovascular, renal and many other areas, there is a need to extend expert knowledge. These challenges rely upon a working familiarity with mental illness and with its management.

The fundamental clinical skill of medicine is acquiring the history of the illness from the patient. The patient is the one suffering, they know their symptoms and the doctor's task is to extract this knowledge and expertly interpret it. The history provides the information on which diagnostic hypotheses are formulated. The definitive diagnosis is determined from the differential diagnoses with the assistance of objective information provided by the clinical examination and the investigations. Acquiring a psychiatric history is little different to any other medical history. Providing the patient with the opportunity to describe his symptoms, to reveal his narrative, is the key to good history taking. The interrogative pronoun which ensures a description of ill-health is 'how'. 'How is your health affecting you?', 'how are you feeling?', 'how do you toilet?', followed by repeated requests to further describe and elaborate, provides copious information, and more efficiently than with closed questions. Allowing the patient the first half to two-thirds of the interview time for this is appropriate and efficient. The doctor assumes control for the final portion in order to further clarify any details and ask specifically about medications, allergies and personal habits. This interview format applies equally to a full 50-minute psychiatric assessment and a 10-minute general practice consultation. Terminally ill patients are certainly not an exception. Their symptom load and appreciation of the preciousness of time encourages productive history taking in a brief period. Often 10–15 minutes is sufficient. Specific questions needed to be asked of the terminally ill concerning fatigue, hallucinations and suicide risk, for these symptoms tend not to be volunteered.

What constitutes an adequate mental status examination in the dying should be influenced by what the examiner hopes to confirm. Delirium, depression, anxiety and cognitive dysfunctions are the common mental health problems of the dying. Time is limited, for energy and ability to co-operate are compromised. The bare essentials of a mental status examination in a terminally ill patient should include estimates of consciousness, orientation, recent memory, simple calculation and mood. Physical examination of the terminally ill is predominantly a psychological exercise. While academically it is gratifying to confirm the historical impression of an enlarged liver or bronchopneumonia, rarely does this influence a management plan. Most persons have a belief that medical examination, rather than history, is the key to medical practice. Until physically examined, even if the examination is only cursory, most don't consider they have been properly assessed. The stethoscope and the percussion hammer are powerful tools of comfort. This is not to suggest that a medical examination doesn't provide useful confirmatory information, including for mental illness. The traditional medical history and examination is a better assessment tool than the multitude of scales and psychometric measures available.

The practice of clinical psychiatry, and medicine in general, requires knowledge of psychology. Personality traits, coping skills, general intellectual function and current stressors impact upon adjustment to, and living with, terminal illness. Modern psychology is cognitive and behavioural in philosophy. Psychodynamic conceptualisation is less emphasised. There is a considerable literature concerning psychology and severe illness. The psychiatric literature is less robust. The discipline of psychiatry encompasses both organic and psychological dysfunction. The vast majority endure a sad and unfortunate terminal illness with courage and stoicism. They manage 'normally'. For them, psychiatry has nothing to offer. For those with dual pathology, good psychiatry and good palliative medicine can enhance the quality of remaining life.

References

1 Whittier JG. Quoted in MB Strauss (ed). *Familiar Medical Quotations.* Boston: Little, Brown and Company; 1968, p. 578.
2 Cherny NI, Coyle N, Foley KM. Suffering in the advanced cancer patient: a definition and taxonomy. *J of Palliat Care.* 1994; 10: 57–70.
3 Cassel EJ. The nature of suffering and the goals of medicine. *N Engl J Med.* 1982; 306: 639–45.
4 Cherny NI. The treatment of suffering in patients with advanced cancer. In: Cochinov HM and Breitbart W (eds). *Handbook of Psychiatry in Palliative Medicine.* Oxford: Oxford University Press; 2000, pp. 375–96.
5 Finlay I. In: Lloyd-Williams M (ed). *Psychosocial Issues in Palliative Care.* Oxford: Oxford University Press; 2003, p. viii.

Chapter 2

Adjustment and anxiety

The human race is the only one that knows it must die, and it knows this only through its experience. A child brought up alone and transported to a desert island would have no more idea of death than a cat or a plant.

Voltaire (1694–1778)[1]

Dying is a personally unique experience and one that we can not share with another, nor rehearse with any certainty as to how it will be. Yet we know it will happen. 'Never-before-encountered' psychological challenges are presented to the terminally ill.[2] 'Can this be death?' thought the mortally wounded Prince Andrew in Tolstoy's *War and Peace* moments before his death. For many, until they are incurably ill consideration of the psychology and spirituality of death is not contemplated with seriousness. Adjustments and anxieties are inevitably created.

Adjustment disorder (or distress)

Care more particularly for the individual patient than the special features of the disease.

William Osler (1849–1919)[3]

The Diagnostic and Statistical Manual of Mental Disorders (DSM) IV and International Classification of Diseases (ICD) 10 diagnostic criteria for adjustment disorder are imprecise and nebulous.[4] Within 1–3 months of a triggering event, emotional disturbance (marked distress in excess of expected) and behavioural changes (impairment of social/occupational functioning) occur which are not able to be diagnosed as another mental disorder. Anxiety, depressed mood and conduct aberrations are often the prominent symptoms, yet not of the intensity or persistence to meet the specific diagnostic criteria for these conditions. Adjustment disorder refers to someone who is distressed and 'not coping', having recently experienced a stressor, such as a malignant diagnosis, a treatment complication or the awareness of impending death.

Adjustment disorder is reported in 32% of cancer patients, and 35% of cancer sufferers are clinically significantly distressed.[5,6] These would appear to be surprisingly low figures, for at stages it is probable that all cancer patients struggle with their emotions and coping. 'Distress' is not defined in the medical literature. Rather than attempting to differentiate adjustment difficulties from sadness, sorrow, grief, subclinical anxiety, depression and Axis 1 DSM IV diagnoses, it may be more useful to use the term 'distress'. Adjustment disorder may merely be a diagnostic creation to satisfy the American health insurers and permit financial return to health professions. Distress rather than the medical condition of adjustment disorder would avoid psychiatric stigmatisation and acknowledge an expected and normal reaction to an unsettling life event. Risk factors including low ego strength, passive or avoidant coping style, inadequate or inappropriate information, lack of social support, communication problems, treatment-related stressors, number of unresolved concerns and level of partner's distress have been identified.[7] Lack of coping flexibility may well predispose persons to difficulties problem solving and adjusting to the new problems a malignant illness presents.[8] It is difficult to conceive a greater stressor than that of a terminal illness, irrespective of the resilience and resourcefulness of the patient. Indeed those few persons who respond to such illnesses without a behavioural or emotional flinch are probably more likely to suffer significant psychopathology.

Management

There is no empirical research providing information on the most effective treatment of adjustment disorder or its natural course.[9] Possessing appropriate and adequate information, most individuals with the support of their family and social network adjust and adapt. The innate resourcefulness of most is remarkable. Information and empathic (not sympathetic) support provided by the attending medical and nursing staff is surely helpful. Too much complex information, often provided in the modern climate of non-paternalistic medicine, risks enhancing distress and indecision. A fundamental and reassuring task of the health professional is, ironically, to reinforce the normality of distress. Some health professions, particularly psychiatrists, often have little to offer for they are inclined to somewhat trivialise distress or convert it into a medical condition that they think they know how to treat.

Self-help groups may have a role and for some, individual and/or group psychotherapy may be of benefit. Psychodynamic interventions based on a trusting relationship and the relating of earlier experience to the current one is the most effective form of psychotherapy for adjustment disorder.[10] Cognitive–behavioural approaches are however more commonly practised these days. While there is undoubtedly a role for specialist psychotherapists with those struggling profoundly with adjustment distress, the therapeutic costs of making normality into pathology need to be carefully ascertained. The ideal assistance is that provided by the patient's natural support network. Nursing staff are the best-placed professionals to provide support, however specialist counsellors have a role, perhaps an increasing one.

Very short-term and intermittent hypnotic use may be helpful during the crisis period. Insomnia may perpetuate a vicious cycle of distress and fatigue, each amplifying the other. Arresting this cycle can be most beneficial. There is no evidence that antidepressant or antipsychotic medications ameliorate distress. In some communities and cultures alcohol is used. Alcohol is an effective remedy for initial insomnia, until tolerance develops, but it disturbs the sleep architecture and dreams, and fitful awakenings tend to negate the advantage of ease of falling off to sleep. Habitual use and physical dependence can be initiated by an adjustment crisis. Drugs are best avoided, adjustment distress is a psychological process and requires, and is eased by, psychological interventions.

The passage of life is a procession of adjustments to minor and major events. Sadness and distress invariably occur. Such experiences can initiate psychological growth and maturation. Pathological interpretations of adjustment or distress reactions are rarely therapeutic. Distress and cancer are naturally associated. This doesn't mean psychotherapy is not helpful. The illness may be a therapeutic opportunity for both patient and family to sort not only the current, but also older, troubles.

Anxiety states

Acute situational anxiety and panic attacks

The receiving of 'bad news', the discomforts and the humiliations of medical procedures, and the dawning awareness of illness progression are but a few of the predicaments precipitating acute anxiety in the terminally ill. Anxiety commonly increases as disease progresses.[11] It may also be precipitated by the withdrawal of active treatment rendering the patient 'unprotected' or 'abandoned'.[12] The psychological adaptation from curative to palliative care is an anxious phase. The prevalence of pure anxiety symptoms in cancer patients is not established, for often mood symptoms co-exist and panic attacks are presumed to be 'normal'. Lewis in the 1930s proposed a continuum between anxiety and depression and believed they could not be usefully distinguished,[13] an opinion that to this day has not been convincingly refuted.[11] In practice, 'nervous' patients are frequently encountered (*see* Box 2.1). If the anxiety response is very severe and abrupt, it is referred to as a panic attack. Anxiety fades spontaneously and is extinguished, but is easily reactivated by lesser stimuli for some period of time. Somatic symptoms activate the central discomfort, and vice versa, thus a self-perpetuating cycle can be initiated.

Most people at some crisis during their life, such as before an examination or after a frightening occurrence, will have experienced a panic attack. In situations of profound and real danger, panic is rare, rather a sense of calmness and clarity pervades, not unlike its pain equivalent, stress analgesia. Anxiety has a purpose,

---

Box 2.1   Symptoms of anxiety

- *Psychological*: apprehension, panic, inappropriate fear, foreboding, dread, tension, intrusive thoughts of death, catastrophic thoughts, depersonalisation, derealisation, irritability, initial insomnia, impaired concentration, slowed thinking
- *Somatic*:
  - *gastrointestinal*: dry mouth, diarrhoea, indigestion ('butterflies'), anorexia, nausea, dysphagia ('globus hystericus')
  - *cardiovascular*: palpitations, chest ache, tachycardia
  - *respiratory*: hyperventilation ('air hunger'), yawning, sighing
  - *nervous system*: headaches, dizziness, tremor, paraesthesia, shakiness, muscle twitching, restlessness
  - *genitourinary*: urgency, impotence
  - *dermatological*: sweating, rash

like inflammation. Anxiety is the psychic equivalent of pain. It activates the 'fight or flight' response and mobilises the organism to achieve some mastery over the provocative stimulus so it doesn't again disturb equilibrium. Anxiety, like 'stress', functions in constructive and adaptive ways, and indeed psychotherapy utilises this discomfort to incite change. Its essential function is reparative. A little is invigorating but too much is disastrous.

Anxiety may also be pathological. The behavioural consequences, such as fleeing treatment or refusing interventions, may be damaging. Some have a 'trait' propensity to high resting anxiety, thus their threshold is lower. Unprovoked panic is suggestive of it being secondary. Anxiety and panic may be symptomatic of primary psychiatric illnesses such as generalised anxiety, post-traumatic stress disorder or affective disorder. Organic disease creates anxiety. Uncontrolled pain evokes anxiety. Thyroid, parathyroid and adrenocorticotrophic hormone (ACTH)-secreting tumours may cause anxiety. Corticosteroids, respiratory stimulants, drug withdrawal states (included in the elderly diurnal withdrawal symptoms from short-acting hypnotics), neuroleptic-induced akathisia and any major current or impending physiological challenge (such as a pulmonary embolus) may be accompanied by anxiety.[13] Disease of the central nervous system provokes a 'free-floating' anxiety, and in palliative care cerebral tumours and metastases may drive such discomfort independently of any environmental or interpersonal stressors.

Management

Psychological
Verbal reassurances and explanation may not be able to be immediately assimilated because of the cognitive compromise. Touch and stroking may be more effective anxiolytic interventions, and merely the presence of a concerned other may be therapeutic during a crisis. Focusing attention on slow, regular breathing and relaxation serve not only to distract but also to allow carbon dioxide to build up and physiologically check hyperventilation. Breathing into a paper bag is another option, though some can't tolerate the bag over their mouth and nose. Panic is not dangerous – fainting, heart attacks and insanity rarely occur. 'Fighting it' merely prolongs it. Once over the peak, many are ripe to benefit from guidance or interpretation, this being a fundamental tenet of psychotherapies. If the anxiety is persistent, behavioural and cognitive psychotherapies are indicated.

Pharmacological
Medication can allow the psychological interventions to be acceptable to the patient and able to be applied with effect. Medication and psychotherapy are complementary.

Benzodiazepines
The most effective intervention, if the above are not proving effective, is benzodiazepine (BDZ) medication. Benzodiazepines lower overall anxiety and also reduce anticipatory anxiety. For acute anxiety they have greater efficacy than antidepressants, beta-blockers and buspirone.[14] Clonazepam (0.25–0.5 mg)

as oral drops or tablet takes up to 20 minutes to be active, as does lorazepam 0.5–1.0 mg, however subcutaneous midazolam (2.5–5 mg) within moments contains a crisis. The type, dose and route is determined by urgency of the mental state and the preference of the prescriber. BDZs are extraordinarily versatile and can be administered by multiple routes – oral, intranasal, sublingual, buccal, *per rectum* (PR), subcutaneous (SC), intramuscular (IM) and intravenous (IV). If hepatic functioning is severely compromised, oxazepam and lorazepam are renally excreted and therefore a preferable option. The anxiolytic action of benzodiazepines may fade over time and tachyphylaxis may occur (but not invariably), hence the recommendation of short-term use. For most it takes at least several weeks for therapeutic fade to occur. Anxiety, even in crisis, waxes and wanes thus there is continuous variation of dosage requirement, thus encouraging tachyphylaxis.

Other anxiolytics
Buspirone may have a specific role in organic anxiety. Barbiturates remain the ultimate backstop for intractable acute anxiety. Beta-blockers (propranolol 20–40 mg orally) may block the somatic symptoms and interrupt the vicious cycle.

Antidepressant medications
The misnamed antidepressant medications, particularly the selective serotonin reuptake inhibitors (SSRIs), are the most effective long-term medication for chronic anxiety.

Fears

It is faere (fear) I stand most in faere (fear) of.

Montaigne (1533–1592)[15]

The fear of illness and death is universal. The illnesses most feared are those of madness, spinal injury and cancer. Death anxiety is the fear of non-being, of not existing. Surveys have shown 50–80% of cancer patients have concerns or troubling thoughts about death.[16] Death fear is independent of religion and religious practice.[16] Religiosity may camouflage these fears. Spirituality and religious faith may be coping strategies, and perhaps protective ones. Death anxieties may centre on particular concerns such as fears of the manner in which one may die, of life being meaninglessly medically prolonged, of pain and disfigurement, of loss of personal desirability, of being dependent and a burden, of financial and employment losses, of the future care and safety of dependants, and of abandonment by relatives, friends and professional carers. The core theme to these concerns and fears is the loss of control, independence and autonomy associated with the unwanted 'sick and dying role'.

George Washington gave instructions in his will that his body should be kept above ground for three days before burial. Such was Hans Christian Andersen's fear of being buried alive that every night he would place a note on his bed to say that he only appeared to be dead. The fear of being buried alive (taphophobia), a primal fear, is perpetuated by sensational reports of the 'dead' awakening, though is less commonly a fear in the modern world than in centuries past.[17] It stimulated the invention of elaborate warning systems able to be operated from within a coffin, encouraged medical debate on the signs of death and influenced the usual (slow) pace of funeral arrangements. However in cultures and societies in which belief and/or environmental conditions prefer quick burial (by sunset), such fears may be more prevalent. The ponderous ritual of auscultating the chest to certify death is a historic remnant of medicine trying to reassure the living that only when dead will they be buried.

Management

William Heberden (1710–1801) suggested 'physicians ... should disarm death of some of its terrors'.[18] Providing a safe opportunity to express these concerns and fears, education, and reassurance are the core components of management. Gentle exploration of the beliefs and personal experiences that may have re-inforced such fears may be necessary, and for some, more intensive psychother-apy may be required. Because of the novelty of the experience of dying for the individual, the professional alliance with the attending staff, experienced in caring for the dying, may be invaluable. Non-abandonment and the intense desire to contain distress and suffering are crucial staff attitudes. However the primal and fundamental nature of fears about death remains for many, at least to a minor degree.

Phobias

A phobia is an irrational fear of a specific situation. It results in an excessive and unrealistic avoidant reaction to a fearful stimulus. It can't be explained away, though the sufferer recognises it to be an extreme, if not silly, response. Exposure results in panic thus most prefer not to risk this. The commonest simple phobia in oncological practice is needle phobia, a condition that affects up to 10% of the population. The needle puncture triggers an inherited vasovagal reflex of shock and successive needle exposure results in an additional learned reflex.

Phobias may be of doctors, hospices, radiation therapy and chemotherapy. Anticipatory nausea and vomiting (ANV) is a conditioned response to environ-mental cues related to the chemotherapy experience.[11] As chemotherapy courses extend, the intensity of ANV tends to enhance, further reinforcing the phobia. Marcel Proust wonderfully described the sensory cues initiating remembrance (and phobias).[19] The smell of a hospital may evoke fearful memories. Claustrophobia created by the confinement and noise of magnetic resonance imaging (MRI) scanning is not uncommon.

Agoraphobia and social phobia occurring early in the course of illness may delay the seeking of medical care or compromise the attendance at treatment. These pathological conditions lie at the extreme of a continuum from shyness to social avoidance, and are of relevance to 'illness behaviours' for they can adversely influence attendance at the doctor.

Management

Phobias respond well to graded exposure or desensitisation behaviour therapy. Support and explanation are essential components and occasionally background

SSRI or BDZ (or for needle phobia topical anaesthesia) cover is necessary. The weight and demands of disease and treatment may flood the patient, paradoxically resulting in a 'self-cure'.

Benzodiazepines

Much maligned since the early 1970s, benzodiazepines (BDZs) have safely transformed the acute medical management of anxiety. Superior in potency and tolerability to their predecessors such as bromides and barbiturates, their benefits have been underestimated and their risks of dependency overestimated.[14] At low dosage BDZs are anxiolytic, at high dosage they are sedative. Clinically they are easily titrated, however in the mid-range dose (or combined with alcohol) they may cause a state of acute intoxication. It is mainly for these reasons that they have acquired a contentious reputation. The individual BDZs differ in half-life (related mainly to metabolism, not absorption) and potency, though all interact with BDZ receptors and increase gamma-amino butyric acid (GABA) inhibition. Judicious prescribing in the medically ill dictates that the short-acting BDZs should be used. The preference for clonazepam by many in palliative care may be based on history and availability rather than pharmacology.

BDZs are a crucial medicine in the armamentarium of palliative care. They are used as anxiolytic agents, hypnotics, anticonvulsants and sedatives, for acute dyspnoea, delirium tremens, spasm and drug withdrawal states. Though expensive and with a short storage life, there is an antidote available – flumazenil. This has also been trialled therapeutically in hepatic encephalopathy.[20] The concerns regarding potential adverse events of BDZs have probably been overestimated in risk–benefit analyses, certainly at least for the palliative care patient.

Respiratory depression

Parenteral BDZ may induce transient respiratory depression in BDZ-naive persons, as many junior doctors treating prolonged seizures have discovered to their horror. This has not been reported for oral BDZs alone. Sleep apnoea and snoring may be enhanced, and a decrease of the ventilatory response to hypercapnia has been demonstrated.[21] In animal studies, IV administration, and not oral, was required to induce respiratory depression.[22] While the availability of the antidote flumazenil is reassuring, BDZs should be used with caution in the respiratory-compromised patient. Yet in the management of severe dyspnoea this adverse reaction is not problematic unless the dose is deeply sedating.

Dependence and addiction

Physiological dependence, as expressed by withdrawal symptoms (insomnia, tremor, sweating, tachycardia, light sensitivity, optical distortions, depersonalisation, derealisation, nervousness, seizures, delirium), depends primarily on the duration of treatment and the dose of BDZ. Withdrawal symptomatology, which occurs in up to 80% of patients, normally appears only after treatment of more than 4 months' duration,[14] and 2–3 days after abrupt cessation of short-acting

BDZ and 5–7 days after long-acting BDZ discontinuation.[23] Symptoms tend to be more intense with short-acting BDZ withdrawal and clinically need to be distinguished from rebound phenomena, that is the dramatic return of the original anxiety symptoms. There is a distinct emerging trend to maintain that small group of chronic anxiety sufferers who are not responsive to other interventions and who are on BDZs long-term for these disorders tend to be relapsing. Dose escalation tends not to be a problem, nor does fading efficacy, though physiological dependency needs to be acknowledged for these patients. Apart from dependency, there is no evidence of psychiatric morbidity caused by long-term use of BDZ.[24] The risk of addiction and abuse of BDZs increases with duration, dosage, short-action BDZ, severity of symptoms, additional stressors and for certain personality types.[14] Personality disordered persons may be at enhanced risk.[14] Anxious,[24] dysthymic,[14] and borderline[25] personality traits may pose the greatest risk for addiction. Rapid dose escalation, drug seeking and reports of mislaid prescriptions may indicate the emergence of psychological dependence, but this adverse event is unusual in the acutely medically ill. The chaotic drug-dependent patient with recently diagnosed cancer may 'arrive' at palliative care addicted to many substances including BDZs. The more important clinical concern in palliative care is the thoughtless cessation of long-term BDZ prescribed for anxiety or insomnia and the resultant withdrawal symptoms. Gradual tapering of the dose with a view to eventual withdrawal may not be a practical option in palliative care. Administering a longer-acting, maintenance BDZ is usually more feasible and humane in the dying.

Paradoxical behaviours

Disinhibition or aggressive dyscontrol in patients treated with BDZs is uncommon. Dietch estimated the incidence of behaviours such as irritability, verbal hostility and frank assault associated with BDZs to be less than 1%.[26] At-risk persons include the neurologically impaired, the elderly, adolescents, alcohol and substance users, the severe personality disordered and those with pre-existing impulsive behavioural problems.[27] However in a retrospective chart review of 323 psychiatric inpatients (a high-risk group) prescribed either alprazolam or clonazepam, and a control group who received no BDZ, no differences between the groups as to behavioural disinhibition could be found.[27] BDZs may unmask underlying depressive affect; however in the anxious dysthymic they may relieve such symptoms. BDZs are similar to alcohol in that the effects vary with the dose. In the frail terminally ill it is prudent to dose with care and avoid intoxicating mid-range doses.

Amnesia/cognitive impairments

Amnestic disorders have been reported, with high dosage of short-acting BDZs, specifically triazolam and lorazepam. These dose-dependent memory losses principally affect the assimilation of new information into the long-term memory and not memory contents previously learned. Usually the deficit is short lasting and reversible, and with chronic BDZ administration tolerance to memory deficits appears to develop.[28] Lipid solubility may be a factor, clonazepam being the least likely to cause memory impairment.[28] The beneficial use of short-acting high-potency BDZ to abolish traumatic memories of a horrific procedure or medical event, such as awareness during anaesthesia, has been advocated. Combination with alcohol amplifies the risks of neuropsychiatric adverse reactions of BDZs significantly. Tiredness and drowsiness affecting concentration and impairing motor function can occur early in treatment, with high dosage, and particularly in the frail elderly. Interestingly these problems are more detectable in normal subjects than anxious patients. While the sedation may be beneficial at night, it is a dangerous side-effect by day, greatly enhancing the risk of falls and dulling the quality of remaining life. Clinically these risks need to be weighed against the inconvenience and the non-pharmacological hangover of a sleepless night. Untreated insomniacs are more at risk for daytime drowsiness and despondency than those using BDZ hypnotics.[29] Tolerance to the sedating adverse reactions tends to occur; it is less certain if tolerance to the anti-anxiety and hypnotic effects evolves. Metabolic tolerance to BDZs does not occur; at high dose minor functional tolerance may occur.

Post-traumatic anxiety states

Traumatic experiences are sadly a part of life for many, if not most. An American citizen's lifetime exposure to traumatic events shows that the exposure rate to life-threatening illness is 4.7/100, a little less than the risk of being shot or raped, and considerably less than being involved in a motor vehicle accident at 28/100.[30] The normal response to a sudden, unexpected and distressing event is a transient acute stress disorder (ASD). ASD ensures immediate emotional anaesthesia following the trauma and an exaggerated arousal state in order to help survive the crisis. Like grief, over time (and in a safe environment) these symptoms spontaneously resolve, and within 12 months for the majority the troubling symptoms have dissipated. Yet intrusive recollections and nightmares of the event and symptoms of physiological readiness for 'flight or fight' can still be cued by reminders, particularly sensory ones. Some with ASD may develop post-traumatic stress disorder (PTSD) (*see* Box 2.2). PTSD is a disorder induced by fright undermining an individual's sense of safety and exposing their vulnerability and powerlessness. It is a complex biopsychosocial disorder and not merely a psychological reaction to a terrible occurrence. The symptoms of PTSD have adaptive survival purposes until such time as the threat to life has abated, at which stage these persisting symptoms are maladaptive. A cost of modern oncology practice 'converting' cancer to a chronic life-threatening disease is that psychological traumatic opportunities are also increased. While up to 93% of the general population report exposure to traumatic events, only approximately 5–12% develop PTSD.[31] The vast majority of those exposed cope with great fortitude and without ongoing psychological or psychiatric symptoms. The lifetime prevalence of PTSD in the general population is 5–6% of men and 10–12% of women.[32] The probability of evolving PTSD is dependent on the type of trauma (exposure rate/100: life-threatening illness 1.1, rape 49.0), sex, past psychiatric history, prior traumatic history (trauma is cumulative), low education, social status, age and many other factors. The commonest psychiatric sequela of traumatic exposure is depressive disorder.

Box 2.2 Post-traumatic stress disorder

- *Exposure to a traumatic event*: involving the perception of life being threatened
- *Symptoms*:
  - *re-experiencing cluster*: recurrent and intrusive recollections of the traumatic event, recurring distressing dreams and nightmares, dissociative reactions (e.g. flashbacks)
  - *avoidance/numbing cluster*: avoiding thoughts, feelings and stimuli of the event, amnesia for part of the event, detachment, reduced ability to feel emotions
  - *hyperarousal cluster*: anxiety, hyperalertness, insomnia, exaggerated startle reflex, irritability, angry outbursts, poor concentration, safety consciousness
- *duration*: acute <3 months, chronic >3 months

Cancer, particularly at the time of diagnosis, can induce post-traumatic symptoms.[33] Medical diagnoses and procedures may result in extreme fear, helplessness, or horror; these reactions being required descriptors of the DSM IV criteria for a traumatic stressor. The degree of fear of dying is related to the risk.[34] Alter reported that nearly half of a group of cancer survivors reported post-traumatic symptoms, with 4% meeting a current diagnosis of PTSD.[35] Current or past PTSD diagnosis in HIV-positive men was found to be 30%.[36] The likelihood of PTSD is however lower among medical patients compared to, for example, rape victims. Much of the trauma literature concerns young women with early breast cancer where such a diagnosis is clearly catastrophic. As is to be expected, such symptoms are prone to reactivations at various stages through the illness, for reminders cannot be avoided if a hospitalisation or a procedure is necessary.

But not only are the rates of post-traumatic symptoms low following medical illness, the symptoms that evolve tend not to be typical of classical PTSD. The precipitating stressor, the illness, is not 'man-made' or involving interpersonal violence, though medical complications may be perceived to be. Naturally occurring stressors and disasters are less intense stressors and generally illness, even if contributed to by risky behaviours such as smoking, excessive use of alcohol and extreme sun exposure, are interpreted by most as 'fate' or misfortune. An ongoing treatment-related stressor can be prepared for and should take place in a supportive environment, features that further mute helplessness and horror. The intrusive thoughts, dreams and nightmares of these patients are often future-orientated.[33] They may concern fears of relapse, mutilation, pain and dying. They are not the repetitious, recurrent recollections of the traumatic event of classical PTSD. In fact they are more typical of pervasive worry and anxious apprehension of generalised anxiety disorder.[33] Neither are the sympathetic nervous system-driven arousal symptoms and signs associated with the intrusive thoughts so evident. Medical events are more prone to induce chronic anxiety than post-traumatic states such as ASD and PTSD.

Victims of severe trauma such as Holocaust survivors, Indochinese boat people, displaced refugees and war veterans require particular consideration. The diagnosis of a fatal illness and associated re-exposure to dying may reactivate earlier close-to-death experiences. The pain and cachexia of advanced cancer serve as vivid reminders of torture or starvation, and the loss of control over destiny undermines active coping strategies and the conscious memory suppression that had allowed at least a semblance of quality of post-traumatic life.

Management

Ensuring safety, rest and sleep, medical stabilisation, allowing patients to 'tell their story' (but only if they have a need to) and providing an emotionally warm and supportive environment is necessary 'emotional first aid'. The critical ingredient is the retention of the victim's remaining personal competency and coping strategies, to allow rapid regaining of some control and dignity.[37]

In acute traumatic situations, critical incident debriefing and reworking (cathartic/exposure) therapies have been shown to increase the risks of PTSD,[38] though they may be therapeutic for ASD. Indulgent and vicarious interest in the trauma story may be as damaging as blatant disinterest. Minimising the distress and secondary sequelae (secondary prevention) is important in preventing persistence of symptoms. Psycho-education, psychological interventions (e.g. relaxation techniques, cognitive–behavioural therapy), pharmacological anxiolysis (short-term benzodiazepines, opioids, SSRIs, alpha$_2$-adrenergic blockers, beta-blockers) and the pursuing of ongoing interest and attention in the person and their experience are all of therapeutic value for those traumatised by their illness and/or its treatments. Initial use of a hypnotic agent, followed up after 3 weeks (if necessary) by an SSRI has been recommended for acute persistent PTSD symptoms in primary care.[39]

ASD has an excellent spontaneous recovery rate, as has acute PTSD, for 60% have been shown to remit spontaneously within 6–12 months.[40] But once chronic, PTSD is notoriously difficult to effectively treat. As yet, preventing PTSD is not possible. Palliating its symptoms is often achievable by combinations of psychotherapy and pharmacotherapy. Assertive management of co-morbid conditions such as major depressive illness and substance misuse (perhaps initiated as self-treatment) is important. Establishing a therapeutic alliance with the traumatised is difficult. Even the grave symptoms of terminal illness and attentive care may not persuade the patient to trust in another. The multidisciplinary care provided, the distractions of physiological symptoms of malignant disease, and psychotropic medications can in combination sometimes overcome these barriers and allow a belated therapeutic opportunity for the sufferer of trauma.

Post-traumatic growth

> As the strength of the body lies chiefly in being able to endure hardships, so also does that of the mind.
>
> John Locke (1632–1704)[41]

Psychological development, maturation and 'growth' can be precipitated by difficult and traumatic events, such as severe medical illness. This phenomenon has long been recognised in philosophy, literature and religion.[42,43] Some patients consider themselves 'better persons' consequent upon this experience. Improved interpersonal relationships, an enhanced sense of spirituality and a greater purpose in life, in patient and partner, are examples of such changes.[44] Estimates of the prevalence of these consequences range from 40% to 70%.[44,45] Stable pre-cancer personality and social functioning are predictive factors. There is a consistently linear relationship between the degree of trauma and growth.[43] Greater stress related to the illness and greater perceived risks to life are associated with adversarial growth.[45] The precipitating event is required to be 'seismic', sufficient to shake basic assumptions about the self and the world.[46] Post-traumatic growth (PTG) can be accompanied by post-traumatic stress symptoms, however the aetiological stressors in PTG and PTSD differ. Fear may induce cognitive and behavioural change, fright can result in negative sequelae including PTSD.[47] If illness psychologically shakes rather than startles an individual's world, it can be a positive psychological event.

References

1 Voltaire. Quoted in: DJ Enright (ed). *The Oxford Book of Death*. Oxford: Oxford University Press; 1983, p. ix.
2 Cochinov HM. Psychiatry and terminal illness. *Can J Psychiatry*. 2000; 45; 143–50.
3 Osler W. Address to medical students. *Albany Med Annals*. 1899; 20: 307–9.
4 Passik SD and Kirsh KL. Anxiety and adjustment disorders. In: Lloyd-Williams M (ed). *Psychosocial Issues in Palliative Care*. Oxford: Oxford University Press; 2003, p. 72.
5 Derogatis L, Morrow G and Fetting J. The prevalence of psychiatric disorders among cancer patients. *JAMA*. 1983; 249: 751–7.
6 Zabora J. Screening procedures for psychosocial distress. In: Holland J (ed). *Psychooncology*. New York: Oxford University Press; 1998, pp. 653–61.
7 Walker L, Walker M and Sharp D. Current provision of psychosocial care within palliative care. In: Lloyd-Williams M (ed). *Psychosocial Issues in Palliative Care*. Oxford: Oxford University Press; 2003, pp. 49–65.
8 American Society of Psychosocial and Behavioral Oncology/AIDS. *Standards of Care for the Management of Distress in Patients with Cancer*. New York: American Society of Psychosocial and Behavioral Oncology/AIDS; 1999.
9 Berney A and Stiefel F. Psychiatric symptoms. In: Voltz R, Bernat JL, Borasio GD *et al*. (eds). *Palliative Care in Neurology*. Oxford: Oxford University Press; 2004, pp. 275–6.
10 Guex P, Stiefel F and Rousselle I. Psychotherapy with patients with cancer. *Psychotherapy Rev*. 2000; 2: 269–75.
11 Himmelhoch J, Levine J and Gershon S. Historical overview of the relationship between anxiety disorders and affective disorders. *Depress Anxiety*. 2001; 14: 535–66.
12 Payne DK and Massie MJ. Anxiety in palliative care. In: Cochinov HM and Brietbart W (eds). *Handbook of Psychiatry in Palliative Medicine*. Oxford: Oxford University Press; 2000, pp. 63–74.
13 Lewis A. Melancholia: a clinical survey of depressive states. *J Mental Sci*. 1934; 80: 277–378.
14 Moller H-J. Effectiveness and safety of benzodiazepines. *J Clin Psychopharmacol*. 1999; 19(suppl 2): 2S–11.S.

15 Montaigne M. Of faere. *The Essays of Montaigne done into English by John Florio*. The First Book, Ch. xvii. New York: AMS Press; 1967, p. 67.

16 Cherny N. The treatment of suffering in patients with advanced cancer. In: Cochinov HM and Brietbart W (eds). *Handbook of Psychiatry in Palliative Medicine*. Oxford: Oxford University Press; 2000, p. 385.

17 Bondeson J. *Buried Alive: the terrifying history of our most primal fear*. New York: WW Norton; 2001.

18 Heberden W. *Commentaries on the History and Cure of Diseases*. Ch. 51. Quoted in: MB Strauss (ed). *Familiar Medical Quotations*. Boston: Little Brown and Company; 1968, p. 159.

19 Proust M. *Remembrance of Things Past* (tr. CK Scott Moncrieff). London: Chatto & Windus; 1952.

20 Bostwick JM and Masterson BJ. Psychopharmacological treatment of delirium to restore mental capacity. *Psychosomatics*. 1998; 39: 112–17.

21 Cohn MA. Hypnotics and the control of breathing; a review. *Br J Clin Pharmacol*. 1983; 16: 245S–250S.

22 Sakai Y. Comparative study on the depressive action of several benzodiazepines minor tranquilizers [Article in Japanese]. *Nippon Yakurigaku Zasshi*. 1979; 75: 777–87.

23 Noyes RJ, Garvey MJ, Cook BL and Perry PJ. Benzodiazepine withdrawal: a review of the evidence. *J Clin Psychiatry*. 1988; 49: 382–9.

24 Mattilla-Evenden M, Bergman U and Franck J. A study of benzodiazepine users claiming drug-induced psychiatric morbidity. *Nordic J Psychiatry*. 2001; 55: 271–8.

25 Rothschild A, Shindul-Rothschild JA, Viguera A, Murray M and Brewster S. Comparison of the frequency of behavioral disinhibition on alprazolam, clonazepam or no benzodiazepine in hospitalised psychiatric patients. *J Clin Psychopharmacol*. 2000; 20: 7–11.

26 Dietch JT and Jennings RK. Aggressive dyscontrol in patients treated with benzodiazepines. *J Clin Psychiatry*. 1988; 49: 184–8.

27 Paton C. Benzodiazepines and disinhibition; a review. *Psychiatr Bull*. 2002; 26: 460–2.

28 Chouinard G. Issues in the clinical use of benzodiazepines: potency, withdrawal and rebound. *J Clin Psychiatry*. 2004; 65(suppl 5): 7–12.

29 Balter MB and Uhlenhuth EH. The beneficial and adverse effects of hypnotics. *J Clin Psychiatry*. 1991; 52(suppl 7): 16–23.

30 Breslau N, Kessler RC, Chilcoat HD *et al*. Trauma and posttraumatic stress disorder in the community: the 1996 Detroit Area Survey of Trauma. *Arch Gen Psychiatry*. 1998; 55: 626–32.

31 Lee D and Young K. Post-traumatic stress disorder: diagnostic issues and epidemiology in adult survivors of traumatic events. *Int Rev Psychiatry*. 2001; 13: 150–8.

32 Resnick PA. *Stress and Trauma*. London: Psychology Press Ltd; 2001.

33 Mundy E and Baum A. Medical disorders as a cause of psychological trauma and posttraumatic stress disorder. *Curr Opin Psychiatry*. 2004; 17: 123–7.

34 McFarlane AC. The aetiology of post-traumatic stress disorders following natural disaster. *Br J Psychiatry*. 1988; 152: 116–21.

35 Alter CL, Pelcovitz D, Axelrod A *et al*. The identification of PTSD in cancer survivors. *Psychosomatics*. 1996; 37: 137–43.

36 Kelly B, Raphael B, Judd F *et al*. Posttraumatic stress disorder in response to HIV infection. *Gen Hosp Psychiatry*. 1998; 20: 345–52.

37 American Psychiatric Association Guidelines. Practice guideline for the treatment of patients with acute stress disorder and posttraumatic stress disorder. *Am J Psychiatry*. 2004; 161: 11(suppl): 3–23.

38 Mayou RA, Ehlers A and Hobbs M. Psychological debriefing for road traffic accident victims: three-year follow-up of a randomised controlled trial. *Br J Psychiatry*. 2000; 176: 589–93.

39 Ballenger JC, Davidson JRT, Lecrubier Y *et al.* Consensus statement on post-traumatic stress disorder from the International Consensus Group on Depression and Anxiety. *J Clin Psychiatry*. 2000; 61(suppl 5): 60–6.

40 Kessler RC, Sonnega A, Hughes M and Nelson CB. Posttraumatic stress disorder in the national co-morbidity study. *Arch Gen Psychiatry*. 1995; 52: 1048–60.

41 Locke J. *Some Thoughts Concerning Education and of the Conduct of the Understanding*. RW Grant and N Tarcov (eds). Indianopolis: Hackett; 1996, p. 25.

42 Tedeschi RG and Calhoun LG. *Trauma and Transformation: growing in the aftermath of suffering*. Thousand Oaks, CA: Sage; 1995.

43 Linley PA and Joseph S. Positive change following trauma and adversity: a review. *J Traumatic Stress*. 2004; 17: 11–21.

44 Andrykowski MA, Brady MJ and Hunt JW. Positive psychosocial adjustment in potential bone marrow transplant recipients: cancer as a psychosocial transition. *Psychooncology*. 1993; 2: 261–76.

45 Widows MR, Jacobsen PB, Booth-Jones M *et al.* Predictors of posttraumatic growth following bone marrow transplantation for cancer. *Health Psychology*. 2005; 24: 266–73.

46 Calhoun LC and Tedeschi RG. Posttraumatic growth: future directions. In: Tedeschi RG, Park CL and Calhoun LG (eds). *Posttraumatic Growth: positive changes in the aftermath of crisis*. Mahwah, NJ: Erlbaum; 1998, pp. 215–38.

47 Vaiva G, Brunet A, Lebigot F *et al.* Fright (Effroi) and other peritraumatic responses after a serious motor vehicle accident: prospective influence on acute PTSD development. *Can J Psychiatry*. 2003; 48: 395–401.

Chapter 3

Psychological issues and dying

Bodies devoid of mind are as statues in the market place.

Euripedes (484–406 BC)[1]

Much has been written of psychology and cancer. Putative psychological causative factors, psychology affecting progress and psychotherapy all have a considerable literature. There is less written about psychology in the terminal phase of life.

Psychological responses to illness

An adverse life event, such as an illness, induces emotional responses (e.g. anger, fear, sadness, shame) and behavioural responses (e.g. support seeking, non-compliance, co-operation). These are multidetermined. The characteristics of the disease, life experience, temperament, personality, illness concept, coping styles, and defence mechanisms impact upon the eventual responses.

Personality traits (or disorder, if severe) shape the responses. Every person has a unique character. There are clusters of behavioural styles which encompass most characters (see Table 3.1).[2] Stressors, both psychosocial and physiological, unmask and highlight personality traits, which are often well camouflaged by social customs and manners. Ego defence mechanisms are automatic psychological processes by which the mind confronts the threat (see Table 3.2).[3] They serve to unconsciously rearrange the mental conflict created, and allow 'peace of mind'. They create a protective illusion which can be adaptive and/or pathological.[3] 'Immature' defence styles may be predictive of lower survival rates in cancer patients.[4] Ego defences are mechanisms that retain equilibrium, though potentially at the cost of psychological symptoms. The defence mechanisms used are closely linked to personality and maturity. Cognitive (thoughtful) and behavioural strategies, which are referred to as coping, are also individualistic. Preferred coping styles are personality and experientially learned methods of problem solving and regulating emotional response. Appraisal of the threat and the choice of coping styles are influenced by how the patient considers the illness. Each individual is different in the ways they respond. Responses are dynamic, fluctuating and changing continually.

The emotive responses induced in others by the patient are termed counter-transference (even if the reaction is conscious and self-acknowledged). Professionalism should mute responses on the part of the doctor, and by recognising the process and abiding by simple management guidelines, the patient's illness can be properly attended to (see Table 3.1).

19

Table 3.1   Personality and illness (adapted from reference 2)

Personality trait	Personality characteristics	Meaning of illness	Countertransference response	Management
Dependent	Needy, self-doubting, helpless, demanding, seeking reassurances	Fears abandonment	Flattered initially, overwhelmed, avoidant of patient	Reassure within limits; mobilise others to share dependency; schedule regular, brief consultations
Obsessive/compulsive	Orderly, meticulous, in control, indecisive, restrictive emotions	Loss of control	Admiration, identification, irritation as time-consuming	Encourage collaboration in care; provide medical information; structure and routine
Histrionic	Melodramatic, flirtatious, seeking attention	Loss of attractiveness	Appeal, pity	Firm, clear boundaries; clarify, not confront
Borderline	Impulsive, unstable relationships, identity disturbances, affective instability, self-mutilation	Loss of self	Pity, attraction, saviour	Firm boundaries; shared care; consistency; patience
Narcissistic	Arrogant, entitled, grandiose, vain, indifference to others, devaluing	Shame at loss of self-concept of perfection and invulnerability	Anger, inferiority, prestige of caring for important patient	Foster and sooth battered self-esteem; don't challenge entitlement; empathise with affective emptiness
Paranoid	Suspicious, litigious, distrustful, moralistic, blames others	Proof that the world is against them and medicine is exploiting them	Anger, medicolegal wary and defensive practice, conservative decision-making	Courtesy, honesty, respect; counterprojective dialogue (acknowledge resulting feelings, not the content of ideations); litigious awareness
Antisocial	History of antisocial behaviours, plausible, exploitative, angry	Loss of status, aloneness	Fear, anger	Firm management guidelines; operate in a safe environment
Schizoid	Aloof, distant, eccentric, isolated, socially awkward	Fear of intrusion, interference	Difficult to engage, abandon	Respect privacy; maintain consistent quiet interest

Table 3.2   Ego defence mechanisms (adapted from reference 3)

Defence type	Characteristics	Consequences
Mature defences	Suppression Altruism Humour Sublimation Anticipation	Healthy, admirable defences
'Neurotic' defences	Repression Displacement Reaction formation Intellectualisation Rationalisation	Self-harmful defences (causes personal suffering)
Immature defences	Denial Splitting Idealisation Devaluation Projection Projective identification Acting out Passive aggression	Harmful to others (and indirectly to self), typically used in borderline, narcissistic personality disorders

Denial

Denial, an emotion-focused coping mechanism, occurs when an external reality is too unpleasant to face.[5] Denial is unconscious and aimed at an external threat or an intolerable internal threat. Severe denial occurs in 10% of hospitalised patients with advanced cancer, with more moderate levels of denial occurring in 18%.[6] Denial is not avoidance, which is a voluntary effort to shun the circumstances that bring stressful information to the fore, nor is it suppression.[7] Suppression is a conscious or semiconscious process in which the defence is directed toward an intrapsychic event.[7] Denial can be a normal or pathological response. It may reduce anxiety and promote optimal functioning, while also providing time to more properly assimilate acutely presented catastrophic information. Alternatively it may deprive a patient of treatment opportunities. It has temporal variability and is not an 'all or none' phenomenon.[5] Weisman considered that there are three orders of denial used as defences: denying the primary facts of the illness (the symptoms); denying the inferences to be drawn from the symptoms; and denying the possibility of existence, of death being the end of existence.[8] The illusion of health is eventually dismantled by the symptom burden, particularly pain. Relinquishing second-order denial ('this illness will not overcome me') is the crisis of the poor-prognosis oncology patient. The denial tends to be reinforced by the culture of modern medicine as curers, and the hopes of family. These affirmations are usually more entrenched than those of the individual. The transition from oncology to palliative care involves the difficult process of accepting no prospect of cure. Letting go of all denial and confronting the meaning of one's existence is not tackled by many.[9]

Providing that adequate and comprehensible information has been given, denial has a psychological function. Few are psychologically strong enough to be never in denial through the course of illness. The clinician needs to determine this function and decide if the denial is currently beneficial or harmful. Attentive listening and observing behaviours and attitudes (which may be more revealing than words) allow a clinical judgement to be made. Cognitive strategies that will allow the patient to relax denial involve the titration of reality at quantities able to be coped with. Assertive confrontation merely reinforces for the patient the need to be sheltered from this awful information, and the denial strengthens. A pragmatic, problem-solving approach, allowing the patient to retain a perception of control, and not insisting that they abandon this psychological survival strategy, is the most likely to allow movement. Negotiating a partial, but predominantly beneficial, solution, for a specific time, may unlock the denial. Subsequent similar endeavours may keep the door open. Relinquishing denial is a positive, personal act, not something that can be imposed.[9] Psychological changes and growth can proceed. Transcendence and spirituality are kindled, particularly if the patient approaches the quandaries of the meaning of life by surrendering all denial.[9]

Healthy denial can be a marker of depression and CNS impairment.[6] Healthy denial requires competent cognitions. The lack of self-perception of deficits, and the tendency to strive for an undisturbed state by shrinking the environmental milieu (the death feint) caused by destructive nervous system lesions are automatic survival strategies.[10] Communication is abandoned. Management needs to accept organic denial as being impenetrable.

Hope and hopelessness

> I really believe there is scarcely a greater worry which individuals have to endure than the incurable hope of their friends ... attempting to 'cheer' the sick by making light of their danger and by exaggerating their probabilities of recovery ... The fact is, that the patient is not 'cheered' at all by these well-meaning, most tiresome friends. On the contrary, he is depressed and wearied.
>
> Florence Nightingale (1820–1910)[11]

There is no universal meaning of hope. Hope is considered the confident yet uncertain expectation of achieving a future good which is a realistic possibility.[12] Hope is essential to life. The idea of hope is generally perceived in positive terms.[13] It is multidetermined. Hope is contingent on the ability to find continued meaning in day-to-day existence. Hope is a dynamic, which can be influenced by others, events and the interpretation of these. Hopes do change over a lifetime and through an illness. Hope wards off anxiety and fear, and it can be a protective shield.[13] Fostering denial may allow hope. False or unrealistic hopes are secured by denial and may be presented as hope by healthcare professionals, patients and families.[9] Hope can be propped up by unrealistic information and promises, though such foundations are shaky. False hope can be as devastating as no hope. Denying reality and persuading a positive attitude risks burdening an already vulnerable patient with false optimism. Realistic hope can provoke solace in those who are seriously ill.[13] Reality is a prerequisite for hope.[9] Only by confronting the ambiguities and unfairness of human existence can hope emerge.

Hope entices different, alternate and creative cognitive and emotional processes, thereby allowing ongoing existence, different because of the change in health status, but still rewarding. Realistic or authentic hope is thought to have the potential to change human existence for the better without reaching for the unattainable.[14]

The relationship of hope to emotional status is intimate.[15] Depression sours the ability to hope, pain distracts from the prospect, and delirium destroys any possibility. Those with mature defence mechanisms may cope better if hope is low (and realistic). Those with personality vulnerabilities are further damaged by a lack of hope.[16] Hope can be undermined with both harmful and therapeutic consequences. Fromm identified three behavioural responses to the shattering of hope: persons resign themselves to their fate, they isolate themselves from others and there can be destructiveness.[17] Many suggest that hope should never be destroyed, hence an excuse for not telling patients the truth. Surrendering hope can be beneficial. The existential view is that by recognising the finality of life, the appreciation of the present becomes enhanced. The trivialities of life can be ignored. The poet Theodore Roethke wrote 'in a dark time, the eye begins to see'.[18]

Encouraging realistic hope so the patient can then live whatever life is left to the full may require professional assistance. The refocusing of hope from what is no longer possible to what is more immediately important to the patient and family is considered a fundamental therapeutic task of palliative care. Fostering and strengthening hope is an important nursing task.[13] For hope to be generated in someone, they need to feel loved, cared for and important. It is generated from within and sustained by others. Others, such as nurses, by 'being' with rather than 'doing' for the patient, may convey an attitude that sustains constructive hope.[19] The psychological massaging of hope is a core task of palliative care, but this does not necessarily mean strengthening the hope. Reframing hope may eventually result in surrendering hope. Mature ego defences, good psychological health and 'mature hope' tend to be cited as prerequisites for being able to contemplate the 'depth work' necessary to address that death may be the absolute end of existence. An intent of palliative care is to position the patient so they have the option of letting go and exploring the ultimate mystery. Religion may provide a framework of support for this spiritual adventure.

Withholding medical information is not favoured by patients who value autonomy and a role in medical decision making. Honest communication is the norm in the West. Fears of depriving the patient all semblance of hope by 'truth-dumping' is how this practice is still viewed in many cultures. Family (and the colluding medical establishment) assumes the role of carrying the bad news. Providing information with empathy and consideration usually is paradoxically reassuring to the patient. Ill persons are aware of their symptom load, and ignorance tends to enhance rather than mute fears. In unfamiliar territory, most minds, for reasons of self-preservation, consider the worst predicament, not the safest.

Hopefulness has positive connotations of expectation, possibility and goodness. Hopelessness is not only the deprivation or absence of hope, it is profoundly negative. Dismal, despairing and moribund, the hopeless struggle to survive. Demoralisation is a psychological conceptualisation of hopelessness (*see* Chapter 6). It may be the loss of primordial or fundamental hope. The hopeless do not have the capacity to hope, but being without hope does not necessarily equate with being hopeless.

Regression and idealisation

How sickness enlarges the dimensions of a man's self to himself! He is his own exclusive object.

Charles Lamb (1775–1834)[20]

The 'dying role,' in contrast to the 'sick role', forces prolonged and profound dependency and reliance on others.[21] Independence is lost and control and autonomy challenged. Lying helplessly in bed amplifies this sense of redundancy. There is need to literally 'hang from' others as physical frailties rob the ability to competently self-care. Dependency differs from attachment. The former increases as death approaches, the later dissolves. Attachments are initially activated by serious illness, though progressively are shed.[22] It is appropriate to be dependent at times in life, and dying is such an occasion. In response to the threat of annihilation, regression to previous levels of functioning occurs. The intent is to reorganise and then re-establish the self, 'regression at the service of progression'.[23] It is not possible for the incurably ill to rejuvenate. The ensuing state of more primitive functioning persists.

Regression refers to experiencing the emergence of past, often infantile, trends where such trends are thought to represent the reappearance of modes of functioning that had been abandoned or modified.[24] It can be transient or permanent, slight or severe, and normal or pathological. Aging *per se* does not result in psychological regression, it is dependency that compels this.[25] 'Degenitalisation' of emotional relationships and a more pronounced interest in the oral and anal occurs.[22] The dying patient progressively sheds attachments with others, to focus exclusively on an 'allusory mother'. This psychological object becomes the caregiver. The retrenchment to 'primary narcissism' has consequences. Increased sensitivity and reactivity to emotional events is balanced by the psychological soothing provided by carers.

Along the path to this state of regressive infantile existence, memories of childhood re-ignite. For most these are pleasurable somatic memories. Laid before the development of language these memories are sensory, predominantly olfactory and tactile. 'A dying man, they say, is supposed to see his whole life unfold before him ... in comas I imagined I was home again. I would run up and down the red gypsum hills of my childhood, feeling the dry Oklahoma wind brushing against my cheeks ... the warmth of the extra blanket laid across me in the night, my mother's face.'[26] With regression also emerges the fear of abandonment. Narcissism is a fragile state. In Kleinian terms, the 'good' is exaggerated to overcompensate for the 'bad', which is the fear of rejection.[27] The infant splits off the bad aspects, and they are warded off by denial.[27] Any fear is projected or shifted onto the idealised mothering object. Deeper regression relieves this concern. The very primitive self has few if any relationships and no concept of death. Thus it can experience no losses, or fears. Its experience of pain is reflexive and devoid of the affective and cognitive components of pain. Gratification is oral and satiation of needs simpler. The psychoanalytic theory as represented by Deutsch is:

> when organic activity is coming to an end ... the sources of the impulses and instincts must also begin to run dry ... life-instincts and death-instincts alike

grow weaker, and, since they grow weaker simultaneously, the conflict between them subsides of itself. The fear of death becomes superfluous, no danger is signaled, there is no need for anxiety as a protective warning.[28]

Fusion with 'mother' is comforting.

Tranquility in the face of death ... they have detached themselves from object-relationships to this world, and put their trust in another world, a beyond. Freed from the menace of the superego.[28]

Psychoanalysis intentionally facilitates regression to allow a therapeutic opportunity to rework developmental issues. 'The couch' is used as a trick to encourage regression. Its emphasis is on emotions and not primarily cognitions. Similarly in the dying when talking is no longer sustainable, 'good enough' mothering (multidisciplinary caring) may provide such opportunities. The therapy becomes 'play therapy' in which the therapeutic tools are not toys but the everyday tasks of life. Showering, toileting and making a patient comfortable are physical as well as psychological interventions for the dying. Dependency and regression have evolved pejorative connotations. Understanding the functions of these psychological mechanisms allows them to be therapeutically exploited. Infantile dependency upon others who dominate and provide, creates idealising relationships with those who feed and protect. Palliative care workers are often idealised by their patients. The desperate, regressed patient copes by placing faith in a parental figure, hoping for care and protection. A dying psychiatrist wrote 'like a child, I felt no shame at being bathed ... dependency fears disappeared'.[29] His nurse 'knows everything; in a world that has become my universe, she looms very large'.[29]

A therapeutic alliance was considered by Freud to be 'an effective positive transference'[24] and Fenichel used the description 'a rational transference'.[24] Modern conceptualisation would refer to idealisation rather than transference in this context. Transference is a repetition of past experiences, inappropriate to the present.[24] Freud considered it a 'false connection' between a person who was the object of earlier (usually sexual) wishes and the doctor which results in substantial obstacles to treatment.[24] This can occur during the final phase of life, though the clinical relationship with palliative medicine is brief and barely sufficient to start fermenting a transference relationship. Regression certainly accelerates transference. Cognitive impairment limits transference establishing. More likely it is the oncologist and not the palliative medicine doctor who may be presented with glimpses of such interactions. Transference affects may be positive and negative. The intense rage that the oncologist cannot, or will not, save the patient may be wrapped in transference.

Parallel psychological reactions may be occurring in the supporting family. It is in family members where transference issues may eventuate, often unbeknown to the practitioner. At grief follow-up reviews these issues may surface.

Appearance and body image

A distorted body image or self-impression of our appearance is normal.[30] There is a discrepancy between image and reality. To see oneself in a photograph or a video, to hear a tape-recorded message of one's voice, is not exactly as expected. Most however have reasonably accurate images of physical status and attributes.

The self-image is the core on which the sense of one's identity is built.[31] No baby is perfect, except hopefully to his 'good enough' mother. The child relates to his body in the same way in which his mother relates and related to it. These psychological processes evolve early, within the first 2 years, but continue to develop with the evolution of language and communication until age 7–8 years. Self-love and self-esteem rest on a positive self-image. The ego has primarily a bodily frame, though its creation is multidetermined. The body image is constructed out of the physical body that one has, and the experience with others that this body has.[32] The body image becomes the self-image through the process of identification.[32]

Cachexia and the mutilating consequences of cancer savagely assault body image. If fickle, as in adolescents and severely personality disorder patients, the body image and self-esteem are challenged. Psychological regression enhances this fragility. Culture and fashion influence what is considered to represent beauty, which is usually considered as a visual attribute. Most of the human brain is involved with visual function, and most stimuli are visual. The skin is the largest organ and has the same embryonic origin as the nervous system, hence the intimate relationship between sight and emotions. Illness may fragment the 'psychic envelope' because it shatters the integrity of the physical interface between patient and others.[32] An attractive visual body image helps self-esteem, particularly for women. The desire to be seen, to be looked at, is as inborn as the desire to see.[30] Health and beauty are assumed (incorrectly) to be related. The preoccupation with slimness in the West, in its extreme state anorexia nervosa, is matched by a preference for largeness in most other cultures. Both are only feasible options to the respective wealthy. The slimness of AIDS and cancer is not however appreciated. The most visible physical defects are facial, the focal point of communication. A blemish becomes an 'anchorage point', an ugly head or neck cancer is 'spread' to form an unattractive person.[31] 'You are not looking well' is the most penetrating of health comments. Physical deformity evokes upsetting feelings in others, who prefer to avoid the damaged individual. 'Social death' of the physically unattractive is the extreme consequence. Shunned, shamed and self-conscious, the scared and mutilated struggle to retain composure, dignity and esteem. They fear alienation, rejection, and abandonment, and risk social withdrawal, depression, and loss of identity.

Appearance ceases to be commented upon as the ravages of illness become apparent. The individual avoids the mirror if possible and family learn to collude and not to make mention of how they look. To the nursing and medical staff grossly swollen abdomens and fungating ulcers are usually willingly presented. This necrotic exhibitionism is important communication of physical status, but also challenges psychologically the commitment to care of the staff. Eventually patients may regress 'beyond privacy'. 'There is something in sickness that breaks down the pride of manhood' suggested Charles Dickens (1812–1870).[33]

Disgust and caring

> He was lame, and no-one came near him ... to quiet the raging, bleeding, sore, running, in his maggot-rotten foot.
>
> (Philoctetes) – Sophocles (496–406 BC)[34]

The skin is involved by metastases in 3–4% of malignant tumours. Malignant fungating wounds are unsightly and smelly. They are humiliating and shameful to the sufferer. The practice of palliative care involves acquaintance with disgust.[35] Disgust literally means 'bad taste'. It is evoked by repugnant smell, touch, sight and hearing, and encourages recoil from the offensive stimulus.[36] What constitutes a disgusting stimulus varies among individuals and cultures.[37] Disgust is an emotion, and its function is to support survival by avoiding the dangers of contamination or pollution. It is innate and 'hard-wired'. There is also an alluring component to disgust (e.g. horror movies), as if to keep the response practised.

Caring necessitates overcoming the disgust response.[35] The recoil response can be contained or muted by experience, custom and learning. There are a multitude of coping strategies used such as mouth breathing, dissociative cognitive strategies and intellectualisation. Familiarity eases the shocking revelation. Clinical stoicism is the most important coping strategy. Health professions need to transcend their disgust. To achieve intimacy with another, disgust needs to be suspended. The rewards are considerable, and relationships with these patients are rapidly cemented.[35]

Psychotherapy and the dying

Words are the most powerful drug used by mankind.
Rudyard Kipling (1865–1936)[38]

The assumption that all cancer patients need therapy and that any type of therapy is better than no therapy is unjustified. Psychologically healthy persons do their own psychotherapy. It can be difficult to acquire a developmental history from the dying for practical reasons, but also for the perception of the irrelevance of such history. Identifying those in need of formal therapy can be difficult. Contrary to public impression the vast majority of a population received 'good enough' mothering and have the inherent psychological strengths to manage an incurable illness.

Wrong words and poor therapy have negative side-effects. Psychotherapy undermines personal competency and coping strategies if these are intact and capable. While eventually these initial side-effects can be overcome and surpassed, time is a critical factor in the terminally ill. The relationship with the primary medical caregiver is potentially the most important psychotherapeutic tool.[39] Active listening (listening with concentration, curiosity and empathy) is required. Establishing a relationship, within the context of the delivery of medical care, not only is meaningful for the patient, it bonds them to the management plan. A therapeutic alliance is formed, and psychological healing can begin. Distress is not invariably pathological. It is also deceptive and can be hidden. Assessment of psychological status is necessary, but should not always proceed to therapy. Affirming normality in itself is therapeutic. Non-abandonment, a central ethical obligation for doctors (and all staff), is a core therapeutic component of the professional relationship.[40]

There are as many styles of psychotherapy as therapists, but as infirmity increases, options become more limited. Physical frailty and the inability to sustain attention and concentration enforce the need to shift from formalised, office-based, styles of therapy. The psychological themes remain usually unchanged, though they are often more starkly presented. The value of time increases, and willing patients remove the psychological packaging and protections. Therapies, in general, promote active coping and/or explore emotions.[41] As death approaches insight-orientated therapy is too demanding and time is too limited, cognitive–behavioural models likewise.[41] But components of these may be useful. Group therapies are not feasible. Life narrative therapies addressing the meaning of the illness in the context of the life trajectory, especially if able to be written, are valuable both for the present and for the survivors.[42,43] Existential therapies such as logotherapy and meaning-centred therapy are particularly beneficial for those struggling with morale.[44] Guided imagery can be a short-cut to the psychotherapeutic chase.[45]

With further illness progression, briefer verbal interactions and enhanced physical interactions eventuate. The topics of therapy narrow to the immediate interpersonal relationships and the crisis of the loss of independence. Sensory therapies become increasingly attractive as talking therapies become obsolete. Verbal reassurances can be substituted with touching affirmations. Massage, music, aromatherapy, and 'play' therapies assume importance. They are accessible and consistent with the regressive processes accompanying dying. The practitioners of these therapies, usually nurses, often lack formal psychotherapy training. But skilled and experienced psychotherapists tend not to be able to abandon talking, and neither do they have the flexibility to offer frequent, brief or opportunist psychotherapeutic sessions. The telephone is useful but also limited. Committed therapists de-escalate therapy and continue some supportive contact and liaison with the lead carers. Abandonment is not necessary. Saying goodbye is not the same as 'giving up'.[41] The psychological intuitions of those working with the dying are generally sound. Staff support, supervision and mentoring are valuable for these and indeed all practitioners.

Similar issues concern the psychotherapeutic support of families. The chance emergence of a therapeutic opportunity late at night needs to be addressed by the nursing staff. Formally arranging a family therapy session is bound to be countertherapeutic in such a situation.

Staff burnout

The practice of medicine is demanding and stressful. Inherently no specialty is more or less stressful than any other. The demands of attending patients threatening to die but who usually don't (psychiatry), is as stressful as working with those who know they are dying and do (palliative medicine). The apprenticeship to becoming a specialist is a long indoctrination. Gaining experience of medicine and the medical lifestyle is a rigorous process. Doctors select or gravitate to work within the specialties where they feel most at ease and function most comfortably. Eventually, as the saying goes, a doctor inherits the practice he deserves. All need holidays, and all workers tire and eventually burn out. The symptoms of burnout are low-grade anxiety and affective ones, the consequences are that work performance and enthusiasm falter. Rather than considering the intrapsychic issues, the situational ones (i.e. the work) are conceptualised as aetiologically relevant, hence the term 'burnout'. While this may remove the stigma of psychiatric illness and highlight the need for 'time off', it does not alter the required management of the individual.

Compassion (the work of healing and assisting) fatigues, life outside of work is packed with life events, and collegial relationships are rarely always smooth. Though increasingly medicolegally high risk, and tiresomely bureaucratic, medicine remains a fascinating and usually rewarding occupation (or vocation). Losing control of workload and professional autonomy, challenged by managerial interference, are the most irritating and destructive aspects of the modern consultant's job. These stressors are more prone to inducing burnout than clinical issues and demands. Hardiness is a valuable personality characteristic and a necessary professional attribute.[46] In palliative care practice patients die, mutidisciplinary teams fight, and each day distraught patients and families require empathy and understanding. Caregiving is demanding. Working within personal and professional boundaries is protective and preserving of the practitioner. No-one is immune to burnout, but neither should it be expected or anticipated because one works with the dying. Rates of burnout in palliative care, possibly about 25%, are lower than in other specialty areas.[47] This is probably due to the higher profile of this consequence of dedication to work in palliative care.

References

1　Euripedes. Electra, 386. Quoted in: MB Strauss (ed). *Familiar Medical Quotations.* Boston: Little, Brown and Company; 1968, p. 39.

2　Groves MS and Muskin PR. Psychological responses to illness. In: Levenson JL (ed). *The American Psychiatric Publishing Textbook of Psychosomatic Medicine.* Washington DC: American Psychiatric Publishing; 2005, pp. 67–88.

3　Vaillant GE. *The Wisdom of the Ego.* Cambridge, MA: Harvard University Press; 1993.

4　Beresford TP, Alfers J, Mangum L *et al.* Cancer survival probability as a function of ego defense (adaptive) mechanisms versus depressive symptoms. *Psychosomatics.* 2006; 47: 247–53.

5　Dein S. Working with the patient who is in denial. *Eur J Pall Care.* 2005; 12: 251–3.

6　Cochinov HM, Tataryn DJ, Wilson KG *et al.* Prognostic awareness and the terminally ill. *Psychosomatics.* 2000; 41: 500–4.

7　Chaturvedi SK, Chandra PS. Dealing with difficult situations. In: Chandra PS and Chaturvedi SK (eds). *Psycho-oncology: current issues.* Bangalore: NIMHANS; 1998, pp. 17–20.

8　Weisman A. *On Dying and Denying: a psychiatric study of terminality.* New York: Behavioral Publications; 1972.

9　Hegarty M. The dynamic of hope: hoping in the face of death. *Progr Palliat Care.* 2001; 9: 42–6.

10　Goldstein K. *The Organism.* New York: American Book Co; 1939, pp. 39–56.

11　Nightingale F. From *Notes on Nursing.* In: Downie RS (ed). *The Healing Arts: An Oxford illustrated anthology.* Oxford: Oxford University Press; 1994, p. 237.

12　Default K and Martocchio BC. Symposium on compassionate care for the dying experience. Hope: its spheres and dimensions. *Nurs Clin North Am.* 1985; 20: 379–91.

13　Jones AC. The role of hope in serious illness and dying. *Eur J Pall Care.* 2005; 12: 28–31.

14 Holdcroft C and Williamson C. Assessment of hope in psychiatric and chemically dependent patients. *Appl Nurs Res.* 1991; 4: 129–34.

15 Nekolaichuk C and Bruera E. On the nature of hope in palliative care. *J Palliat Care.* 1998; 14: 36–42.

16 Kwon P. Hope and dysphoria: the moderating role of defense mechanisms. *J Pers.* 2000; 68: 199–223.

17 Fromm E. *The Revolution of Hope: towards a humanized technology.* New York: Harper & Row; 1968.

18 Roethke T. In a Dark Time. *The Collected Poems of Theodore Roethke.* London: Faber and Faber; 1968, p. 239.

19 Kylma J, Vehvilainen-Julkunen K and Lahdevirta J. Hope, despair and hopelessness in living with HIV/AIDS: a grounded theory study. *J Adv Nurs.* 2001; 33: 764–5.

20 Lamb C. The Convalescent. *The Essays of Elia.* London: JM Dent and Sons; 1906, p. 215.

21 Noyes R Jr and Clancy J. The dying role: its relevance to improved patient care. *Psychiatry.* 1977; 40: 41–7.

22 Abiven M. The crisis of dying. *Eur J Palliat Care.* 1995; 2: 29–32.

23 Balint M. Primary narcissism and primary love. *Psychoanal Q.* 1960; 29: 6–43.

24 Sandler J, Dare C and Holder A. *The Patient and the Analyst: the basis of the psychoanalytic process.* New York: International Universities Press; 1972, pp. 37–48.

25 Kimsey LR, Roberts JL and Logan DL. Death, dying, and denial in the aged. *Am J Psychiatry.* 1972; 129: 75–80.

26 Stewart S. *Give Us This Day.* New York: WW Norton; 1999, pp. 234–5.

27 Ploye PM. A note on two important aspects of Kleinian theory 'projective identification' and 'idealisation'. *Br J Psychiatry.* 1984; 145: 55–8.

28 Deutsch F. Euthanasia: a clinical study. *Psychoanal Q.* 1933; 5: 347–68.

29 Morgenstern A, Boverman H and Ganzini L. A psychiatrist in hospice. *Palliat Support Care.* 2003; 1: 89–92.

30 Schider P. *The Image and Appearance of the Human Body: studies in constructive energies of the psyche.* London: Paul Trench Truber; 1935.

31 Bernstein NR. *Emotional Care of the Facially Burned and Disfigured.* Boston: Little Brown and Co; 1976.

32 Madioni F, Morales C and Michel JP. Body image and the impact of terminal disease. *Eur J Palliat Care.* 1997; 4: 160–2.

33 Dickens C. Quoted in: MB Strauss (ed). *Familiar Medical Quotations.* Boston: Little, Brown and Company; 1968, p. 544.

34 Sophocles. *Philoctetes.* In: Grene D and Lattimore R (eds). *The Complete Greek Tragedies* (tr. D Grene). Vol. 4. Chicago: University of Chicago Press; 1957, pp. 401–60.

35 Macleod AD. Disgusting patients. *Prog Palliat Care.* 1999; 7: 299–301.

36 Millar WI. *The Anatomy of Disgust.* Massachusetts: Harvard University Press; 1997.

37 Phillips ML, Young AW, Senior C *et al.* A specific neural substrate for perceiving facial expressions of disgust. *Nature.* 1997; 389: 495–8.

38 Kipling R. Speech, 14 February 1923. In: Knowles E (ed). *The Oxford Dictionary of Twentieth Century Quotations.* Oxford: Oxford University Press; 1998, p. 175.

39 Suchman AL and Matthews DA. What makes the patient-doctor relationship therapeutic? Exploring the connexial dimensions of medical care. *Ann Intern Med.* 1988; 108: 125–30.

40 Quill TE and Cassel CK. Nonabandonment: a central obligation for physicians. *Ann Intern Med.* 1995; 122: 368–74.

41 Rodin G and Gillies LA. Individual psychotherapy for the patient with advanced disease. In: Cochinov HM and Breitbart W (eds). *Handbook of Psychiatry in Palliative Medicine.* Oxford: Oxford University Press; 2000, pp. 189–96.

42 Byock IR. The nature of suffering and the nature of opportunity at the end of life. *Clin Geriatr Med.* 1996; 12: 237–52.

43 Pennebaker JW and Segal JD. Forming a story: the health benefits of narrative. *J Clin Psychol.* 1999; 55: 1243–54.

44 Frankl V. *Man's Search for Meaning.* New York: Washington Square Press; 1959.

45 Kearney M. *Mortally Wounded.* Dublin: Marino Books; 1996.

46 Vachon MLS and Benor R. Staff stress, suffering, and compassion in palliative care. In: Lloyd-Williams M (ed). *Psychosocial Issues in Palliative Care.* Oxford: Oxford University Press; 2003, pp. 165–82.

47 Vachon MLS. Staff stress in hospice/palliative care: a review. *Palliat Med.* 1995; 9: 91–122.

Chapter 4

Pain and psychiatry

Pain is no evil unless it conquers us.

Charles Kingsley (1819–1875)[1]

The management of pain is a basic tenet of palliative care practice. Some of the most complex and perplexing aspects of pain are those factors considered 'non-organic'. Pain, psychiatry and psychology are intimately interconnected.

The experience of pain

Illness is the doctor to whom we pay most heed: to kindness, to knowledge we make promises only: to pain we obey.

Marcel Proust (1871–1922)[2]

Pain is 'an unpleasant sensory and emotional experience, associated with actual or potential tissue damage, or described in terms of such damage'.[3] Pain is what the patient says hurts. This by now well-accepted view highlights that pain is an experiential and emotional symptom. Pain is a 'somatopsychic' experience and its intensity depends both on the extent of tissue damage and on the patient's psychological state. There exists a conflict between the noxious stimulus and the whole individual. Pain, the expression of this conflict, is a viciously 'real' experience for the sufferer. Each individual perceives and portrays pain in an idiosyncratic fashion. There is generally a poor correlation between tissue pathology, disability and treatment response.[4] Women are more sensitive to noxious stimuli than men.[5] Although the threshold for pain in the elderly is not raised, tolerance to perceiving pain is, and they are often diffident asking for pain relief.[6] These factors may partially account for the inadequate analgesic relief offered to the elderly. Cultural, personality and situational influences may enhance expressions of pain or inhibit the behavioural portrayal of pain. Insensitivity to pain, a rare congenital condition, is a major disability for individuals with this disorder are deprived the protection of pain, yet 'stress analgesia', in dangerous predicaments, may be life saving. The physiological clinical signs of pain tend to fade with persistence of pain. Psychological factors are integrated into the pain experience. Uncontrolled pain can mimic psychiatric disorders. It can also aggravate and precipitate mental disorder. Conversely affective, cognitive and behavioural factors have significant influence upon pain.

Pain cannot be measured objectively. Visual analogue scales are the preferred, easiest and best measures of pain. The magnitude of the numerical score has little meaning except when measurements are made serially and comparisons made. Each individual perceives pain uniquely, but over time reasonable consistency and reliability in reporting can be achieved using these scales. Yet defining a meaningful decrease on pain rating scales is difficult. 'Moderate relief' or 'much improved' corresponds to reductions on pain scales of about 30%.[7] Pain rating scales are influenced by many factors including contextual circumstances, disease state, mental status, personality, memory of prior painful states and worries concerning the cause of the pain. The scores tend to be more reflective of the affective and emotional aspects of the pain than of the sensory intensity created by physiological pathology.[8] The clinician adds to this conglomeration of influences with medical knowledge of the painful lesion, experience of how similar pathology in other patients is portrayed and an impression of the situational influences. The resultant clinical estimate of pain is, however, likely to be only approximate.

Adequate pain relief is considered a human right by some advocates. Pain is common. Treatment is generally effective and cheap. Treatment becoming a 'right' may encourage the good clinical and ethical practice that this symptom demands and deserves.

Pain and terminal illness

Pain is a common problem for cancer patients. In advanced disease, 70–90% experience pain, and among those undergoing active treatment at earlier stages for a solid tumour, the prevalence is 30–50%.[9] Adequate relief of pain should be achievable with simple drug regimes in as many as 90%.[9] Undoubtedly considerably improved pain management has been practised in many settings (particularly palliative care) over recent decades. Yet pain remains under-recognised and under-treated in terminal illness.

Acute pain serves to warn the individual of bodily harm and is considered the 'fifth vital sign'. It invites affective, cognitive and behavioural responses designed to result in the relief of the symptom and prevent further tissue damage. Chronic pain has little if any adaptive biological function, and generally is contrary to good-quality functioning. Acute and chronic pains are very different clinical entities. In palliative care, most pains are nocioceptive (or somatic) and 'acute' in the sense that they signal physical damage being caused by the disease. Nocioceptive pain is the cause of as much as three-quarters of cancer pain.[9] Incident pain, pain on movement, can be particularly disabling and erosive to quality of life. Damage to the nervous system by disease or injury may result in neuropathic pain, which is typically described by the patient as being 'burning, shooting and/or stabbing'. Neuropathic pain is often seen in the later phase of many diseases of the peripheral or central nervous system, including malignant disease, AIDS, multiple sclerosis and Parkinson's disease. Such pains tend to endure, even if the original causative factor is removed, and they are difficult to relieve. Neuropathic pains are often centrally represented in the nervous system. The pathophysiological mechanisms of neuropathic pain are multiple, each of which may respond differently to medications, with different mechanisms of action. Partial responses are usually achieved, and polypharmacy is the norm. Response rates with opioids alone, the most effective treatment, are about 50%.[10] The clinical belief that neuropathic pain does not respond to opioids has been disproven.[11] Though less responsive, it is partially responsive to opioids. 'Complete' relief of neuropathic pain with multiple agents may be achievable in 50–60% of research trial patients.[12] In clinical practice, relief of such pain is possible in perhaps only 20–30%. In cancer care invariably the less responsive patients are those suffering neuropathic pains. Visceral pain, caused by neoplastic involvement of internal organs and their nerve supply, may be referred to an anatomical site distinct from the lesion. These pains are difficult for the patient to describe, and are often associated with strong emotional and autonomic responses. Psychosocial factors influence visceral pain, which is probably a variant of (autonomic) neuropathic pain. Psychic or emotional pain is the most perplexing of pains to articulate, conceptualise and manage. Treatment-related pain syndromes are usually neuropathic. Refractory pains are most often incident and neuropathic.

Uncontrolled or poorly controlled pain, in addition to the discomfort felt, may aggravate and/or precipitate psychological and psychiatric symptoms. Similar neurotransmitter changes to those of depression are induced.[13] The neurobiology of pain and depression overlap. Misery and desperation ensue. Pain dominates existence and provokes pleading care-eliciting behaviours. Control of pain needs to be of the highest treatment priority in palliative medicine. Not until pain is manageable can the assessment of other symptoms proceed. Clinically it is important to appreciate that the most severe pain is the pain of most immediate concern to the patient. In those with multiple sites of pain, the relief of the most severe pain may highlight other pains, previously quiescent. Pain is rarely static. Pain assessment needs to be continually repeated together with ongoing review and titration of analgesia.

The psychology of pain

> [Pain is] outside the senses and within the passions of the soul.
> Aristotle (384–322 BC)[14]

Pain elicits alarm, anxiety and fear. Anxiety amplifies the pain experience. Anxiety is an internal process, whereas fear is a response to an external threatening stimulus. Patient identification of initiating or aggravating influences on their pain results in protective avoidance behaviours. These include presenting for medical assistance, if the patient has knowledge that the doctor may have effective therapies, and avoiding any activity that may provoke further pain. Expecting and anticipating pain reinforces this behaviour. Patients with greater pain-related anxiety tend to overpredict new pain.[15] Progressive demobilisation and deactivation result. Fear of moving the neck leads to disabilities such as muscular reactivity, deconditioning and guarded movement of the neck (kinesiophobia). Thus a vicious and ultimately counterproductive cycle is established. Not only is the conditioned stimulus avoided (thus this behaviour cannot be extinguished), but sympathetic nervous system arousal further lowers nociceptive thresholds. Hypervigilant and physiologically stressed, the individual struggles to maintain control. Anxiety seldom occurs in isolation, and depression is highly likely to further contaminate this response. While this phenomenon is particularly well described in chronic non-malignant pain, it is also a typical response to chronic cancer pain. Pain entices a cognitive response. Pain has meaning. Increased levels of pain may be believed by the patient to be caused by spread or recurrence of cancer. This belief has been shown to result in more intense pain than when the pain is believed to be caused by other factors.[16] Catastrophic thinking, the amplification of threatening information, intensifies distress, pain and self-perceived disability. Negative thoughts about personal or social competency increase pain intensity and emotional distress.[17] Pain challenges personal coping and can easily unsettle psychological equilibrium.

In response to an unpleasant stimulus, 'manipulative' behaviours are evoked in an attempt to ward off the unwelcome sensory experience. Anger may erupt. This response is reported in 70% of chronic pain patients, and is directed at the self in 74%, and healthcare professionals in 62%.[18] Anger is not necessarily hostile and goal-directed aggression. It may be verbally expressive and explorative of options as to how the pain may be relieved. It can direct appropriate and culturally acceptable strategies of eliciting the required healthcare. Men are more liable to hostile anger, women tend to be more articulate and expressive.[18] Direct and determined help-seeking communication and behaviour should be supported. The manipulation can be creative. When such responses have failed to provide relief, and pain persists (for medicine is unable to oblige), the 'manipulation' can become interpreted as 'manipulative' (in the pejorative meaning of the word).

Concepts of psychologically induced pain have a long history. Freud's case report of Fraulein Elisabeth R in 1892 has been cited as the first 'scientific' report of conversion or psychogenic pain.[19] Freud actually presented the case to illustrate that psychological conflicts could aggravate and maintain the pain of 'rheumatism'. Beecher's brilliant study on wounded World War II soldiers requiring little analgesia, until after the battle, demonstrated 'stress analgesia'.[20] Arousal and distraction can mute pain transiently, but this doesn't make the pain psychogenic. The concept of 'pain-prone' patients in whom psychic factors played a primary role in the genesis of pain,[21] encouraged DSM III (in 1980) to introduce the category 'psychogenic pain', which was renamed 'somatoform pain disorder' in subsequent versions. Pain is however rarely generated and maintained by psychological forces alone.[22] A more reasonable conceptualisation of psychogenic pain is that of psychologically amplified pain of somatic origin. Pain has an organic initiator and psychosocial influencing factors. Saunders introduced to palliative care the term 'total pain', to refer to the multiplicity of psychological, social, bureaucratic, financial and spiritual factors contributing to, and perhaps creating, pain in the cancer patient.[23] Despite 'adequate analgesia', the pain perseveres unaltered. This is a useful clinical concept provided the organicity of the pain is not entirely dismissed. A clinician's response to therapeutic failure can be that of therapeutic nihilism, and the propensity is to project blame onto the patient for the failure of a usually effective intervention. 'Total pain' could represent inadequate clinical and technical expertise, or it can describe a syndrome in which the perpetuating and maintaining influences on a fundamentally 'organic' pain are psychosocial.

The psychiatry of pain

The anxiety and fear induced by acute pain, if the pain continues, are compounded by affective distress, and eventually perhaps affective disorder. A high percentage of those with persisting non-malignant pain become clinically depressed. Conversely, depressive disorder may present with pain, the so-called 'masked depression'. In an international study, 69% of patients with depression presented with only somatic symptoms, of which pain complaints were commonest.[24] At least 50% of those clinically depressed complain of bodily pains.[25] After insomnia, pain is the commonest symptom of depression. Cultural factors do influence the symptoms of depressive illness, and pain symptoms in depressed non-Western patients are more frequently clinically encountered. The causal relationship between pain and depression has long been controversial. 'Pain-prone' personalities in whom a depressive scar is reactivated by pain, or that personal mastery falters under the impact of pain are such propositions. The 'consequence' model is the most compelling, and particularly in cancer patients in whom there may be no prior history of depression. The cause or effect arguments, to the pragmatic clinician are rarely relevant for they don't usually dictate management. The intimate relationship between mood and pain is undoubted and their mutual aggravating influence on each other likewise. Pain can cause depression, and depression can enhance pain.

The neurobiological explanation of this association may be that the descending pathways of pain modulation in the spinal cord utilise monoamine neurotransmitters. A decrease of serotonin and/or noradrenaline in these pathways would relax the central inhibitory control and release the full intensity of the noxious stimulus. Internal stimuli concerning routine bodily functions, such as digestion and heart rate, are normally suppressed from consciousness by descending serotonergic and noradrenergic pathways. This suppression is not constant, rather it acts as a homeostatic regulator by determining whether attention should be directed towards external threats or to sensations coming from within the body. These regulators account for stress analgesia. If the catecholamines are depleted, routine internal sensory input may become disagreeable (and painful), hence the mechanism of the amplification of pain in depression. In addition to the neurophysiological theory, it is important to consider cognitive and behavioural symptoms of depression compounding the situation. A loss of control is initiated by pain, emerging helplessness as relief is not acquired, catastrophic thinking, avoidance behaviours, and brooding hopelessness leading to non-compliance and suicidal thoughts, add to the desperation. Uncontrolled pain is a major factor in suicidal ideation.[26] Severe unrelieved pain erodes the sense of control, and may entice desperate behaviours, including suicide attempts.

Sleep disturbance secondary to the discomfort of pain and the co-existent depressive disorder, further undermines the ability to cope. Reduced sleep quantity and quality correlate with pain, depression and negative affectivity.[27] Sleep is interrupted by pain, and tiredness sabotages coping strategies. Poor sleep is a contributing factor in lowering the pain threshold.[28] Sleep rebound consecutive to sleep deprivation produces an analgesic effect similar to paracetamol or non-steroidal anti-inflammatory drugs (NSAIDs) in volunteers.[28] Not only does insomnia aggravate pain, it may encourage hypnotic and analgesic misuse. Paracetamol is not uncommonly used by the lay public as a mild hypnotic. NSAID use may disrupt sleep by interfering with melatonin levels and body temperature, however these theoretical consequences are likely to be overwhelmed by the analgesic-induced improvement of sleep. Opioids have been traditionally used as hypnotics, mainly due to their (transient) action on kappa receptors. However, opioids and the sedative side effects of tricyclic antidepressants (TCAs) and anticonvulsants may exacerbate pre-existing obstructive sleep apnoea. Sleep disturbance should be a major therapeutic target in pain management.

Psychiatric issues in the management of pain

Psychotherapy of pain

Teasing out cause and effect of a particular psychological variable is clinically neither easy nor rewarding. Pain management needs to incorporate psychological interventions aimed at effect rather than cause. Pragmatic and 'here-and-now' interventions are necessary, rather than analysis of the cause. Explanation, reassurance, cognitive reframing of negative ideation, and refreshing coping strategies using relaxation, hypnosis, mindfulness meditation, and distraction can be of benefit. Reinforcing coping and cognitive reappraisal augments analgesic pharmacotherapies. Analgesic medications are the foundation of cancer pain management. A pill can be of benefit, but a pill and supportive words can be of greater benefit. The nurse is a powerful analgesic. The destructive psychological spiral initiated by a painful stimulus can be checked by short and simple psychotherapy, enhancing the prospects of a better response to medication.

Pharmacotherapy of pain

Opioid analgesics

The analgesic effects of opioids (chemicals with activity similar to opium) typically decrease the distressing affective component of pain rather than the sensation. The pain remains, though many patients acknowledge that following opioids they are less bothered by the unpleasant sensation. Opioids have a pivotal role in managing cancer pain. The 'gold-standard', 'strong' opioid is morphine, an analgesic that provides effective relief in about 75% of pain patients. Nociceptive pain is most opioid-responsive of pains. For neuropathic and visceral pain, opioids are partially effective. Opioids remain the first-line treatment for neuropathic pain.[12] They are comparable to both TCAs and anticonvulsants.[11,12]

History

Opium, the sap of *Papaver somniferum*, a poppy native to the lakes of Switzerland,[29] colonised to the preferable climatic conditions of the Near East over 5000 years ago. The term 'opiate' refers to derivatives of the opium poppy. 'Narcotic' is a legal and not a medical term. Opium was a common component of many cough, cold, diarrhoea, and teething mixtures until the 20th century. The drug was used liberally, often as laudanum (an alcohol and opium solution). Sertürner, in 1806, identified the active ingredient of opium, morphine. It was the invention of the hypodermic needle by Wood in 1853 that made possible the administration of very potent, and dependence-inducing, morphine. 'Soldier's disease', morphine dependency, was common during the American Civil War. It was during the Victorian era that morphine-induced 'euthanasia' became the preferred mode of medical death. The trafficking of opium from India to China by the British had by the mid-19th century created estimates of up to 25% of the Chinese population dependent on the drug, though these high figures are disputed by more recent scholars.[30] From a position of social acceptance, opium came to be propagated as the 'evil drug' of addiction. In Shanghai in 1909 the first international meeting on matters of drug control was convened in response to this rising moral panic. This initiated the dramatic change towards tight and restrictive regulations. Not only did public attitudes alter, doctors developed 'opiophobia', a fear of prescribing opioids. Cancer patients suffered unnecessarily. It wasn't until the emerging hospice movement in the 1950s that the usefulness and safety of morphine for the dying was re-emphasised. The development of sustained-release formulations in the 1980s again refined clinical use. In 1986 the World Health Organization (WHO) analgesic 'ladder' was published.[31] Medicinal availability of morphine remains severely limited in many countries because of the mythology of its abuse, morphine's association with organised crime, and cost. Methadone and other opioids are alternatives in some of these countries, but many cancer victims worldwide still die in pain.

Adverse effects of opioids

All drugs have adverse effects, and opioids are no exception. The opioid receptors in the brain, spinal cord and peripheral nervous system have differing functions. Mu receptors are most important for analgesia but also induce respiratory depression, miosis, gut motility and euphoria. The kappa and delta receptors have some roles in analgesia, but kappa-receptor stimulation leads to psychiatric adverse drug reactions (ADRs). There are many other opioid receptors of as yet uncertain functions. Each individual person has differing and unique opioid-receptor profiles and genetic expression of enzymes responsible for the metabolism of opioids. Opioids to varying degrees antagonise N-methyl-d-aspartate (NMDA) receptors and activate the descending serotonin and noradrenaline pathways from the brainstem. There is considerable individual variability regarding the effects and adverse effects of these medications. Renal failure is a particular risk factor for morphine side-effects, as its very active metabolite morphine-6-glucuronate (M6G) is renally excreted. If used over large wounds, topical opioids

Table 4.1 Neuropsychiatric adverse reactions of opioids

Clinical phenomena or clinical consequences	Symptoms
Lowering level of consciousness	Sedation Sleep disruption Delirium
Cognitive impairment	Slowing of rate of processing
Perceptual impairment	Hallucinations
Psychomotor impairment	Slowing of motor response Myoclonus
Mood alteration	Antidepressant action
CNS toxicity	Tolerance Hyperalgesia
Dependency Withdrawal syndrome Addiction	

may even induce systemic effects. The introduction of an alternative and effective analgesic, such as a nerve block or surgery, can cause opioid toxicity if the opioid dose is not appropriately adjusted.

Opioid neuropsychiatric adverse reactions include (*see* Table 4.1):

- *lowering of the level of consciousness (sedation, sleep disruption, delirium)*: opioids commonly cause sedation on initiation and during dose escalation, but tolerance to this usually develops within days. The widespread public belief that 'morphine kills the dying' is related to its narcosing effects. Differing opioids have differing sedating and anticholinergic effects, thus opioid rotation may be an option, as might the addition of a psychostimulant or more gradual dose increments. Opioids suppress rapid eye movement (REM) sleep and to a lesser extent non-REM (NREM) sleep, thus total sleep time and sleep efficiency are reduced.[32] Opioids disrupt sleep architecture and a more fragmented sleep may result, although it is often difficult to establish whether this is attributable to the drug or the underlying disease.[32] Methylphenidate has been shown to improve this sleep disruption.[33] In clinical practice the sedation and analgesia associated with opioids tends to enhance rather than disrupt sleep. It is named after Morpheus, the god of sleep. The incidence of morphine-induced confusion is a few per cent, though recent authors suggest a much higher rate of opioid-induced hypoactive deliria.[34] Opioids are reported to precipitate delirium and cause it.[33–35] Clinically differentiating the precise causes of delirium towards the end of life is not usually possible. Opioids do affect the cholinergic–dopaminergic balance. That this may be commoner with morphine than other opioids may be accounted for by the accumulation of M6G, particularly as renal function falters. The delirogenic potential of opioids may be reduced by opioid rotation or substitution,[36] the introduction of haloperidol, discontinuation of other anticholinergic medications, the introduction of procholinergic medication, or hydration (to increase morphine metabolite clearance). Improvements are recorded in 60–70% with opioid rotation and hydration.[34] Most authors suggest dose reductions of 50–75% on opioid substitution. The reduced dose may be as relevant as the change of opioid.
- *cognitive impairments*: the prevalence of cognitive dysfunction in the terminally ill is very high, particularly as death approaches. Separating disease from drug effects is difficult. In healthy volunteers, parenteral opioids have been associated with significant dose-related cognitive impairments, whereas oral opioids are associated with only insignificant or mild deficits, and even improved cognition.[35] In patients with advanced cancer, little or no deterioration of cognitive performance has been demonstrated when initiated on opioids.[35] Pain is associated with poorer performance on memory testing than treatment with opioids.[34] The rate of processing information, rather than accuracy, is the prominent cognitive impairment with opioids. This is less than with lorazepam.[34] Impairments are greatest with pethidine, less with hydromorphine, less again with morphine, and less again with methadone.[34] The impairments are dose related,[34] and tolerance develops to them within days. In patients with chronic non-malignant pain studies indicate mainly improved cognitions on opioids,[35] except for those on tricyclic antidepressants (TCAs).[37] Many patients on opioids report mental dulling, fuzziness, being more accident prone, making more mistakes and struggling with cognitive

dexterity. The consensus is that on stable oral doses, transient and mild cognitive impairments may occur. Management by dose reduction, opioid rotation, hydration, and with psychostimulants has been proposed. The most effective intervention may be adequate pain relief.[35]

- *perceptual impairments*: while there are numerous anecdotal reports of opioid-induced hallucinations and nightmares, particularly in postoperative settings, disentangling these clinical phenomena from prodromal symptoms of delirium is most difficult. In a study of hospice patients, almost half experienced visual hallucinations, this being more likely in those taking morphine, although this association was not strong.[38] Morphine tends to be 'blamed' for such mental aberrations.

- *psychomotor impairments*: the evidence for an adverse effect of opioids on psychomotor abilities, such as driving, is conflicting. There is no compelling medical evidence that driving is unsafe while taking opioids, provided the dose is stable.[35,39] Long-term use of morphine had only slight effect on driving.[39] A simple bedside test of opioid-induced psychomotor impairment is to ask the patient to tap their finger for ten seconds. Most only manage three taps.

- *mood alteration*: the 17th century English doctor Napier prescribed opiates for 8% of his melancholic patients (and more commonly for his psychotic patients).[40] In 1850, opioids were considered to be specific treatments for melancholia.[41] The 'laudanum cure', especially recommended for agitated depression, consisting of 16 mg tincture of opiate, increased by 3 mg/day for 22 days and then gradually reduced by 2 mg/day, was used up to the mid-1950s.[42] Positive mood effects have been demonstrated in cancer patients treated with opioids.[43] Low-dose buprenorphine has been used to effectively treat refractory depression in seven patients.[41] Long-term use of codeine is associated with, but not proven to be causative of, depressive symptoms.[44] Codeine as an antidepressant has not been shown to be effective.[42] Nalorphine is an inducer of dysphoria because of its kappa-receptor activity.[45]

- *direct CNS toxicity/tolerance*: apoptosis and damage of neural cells by opioids is a major cause of their adverse effects.[46] There may be direct damage to the receptors,[46] or the effect may be because of activation of NMDA receptors.[47] Myoclonus, noted often at high opioid doses, especially in the presence of pre-existing spinal lesions, may be a sign of neurotransmitter aberrations induced by the opioid. Hyperalgesia, 'wind up', is contributed to by the loss of GABAminergic cells within the dorsal spinal cord,[47] and alterations in NMDA and glycine functions.[46] Tolerance to opioids (where the same dose results in less analgesia or an increased dose fails to improve analgesia) in palliative care patients occurs, but is rarely a clinical problem unless the doses are high.[10] Separating tolerance and disease progression clinically is most challenging. Tolerance may be to both analgesia and to opioid adverse effects. Stable dosing regimes suggest it is not a frequent problem, but it has been shown with parenteral opioids.[48] Tolerance to sedation, cognitive impairments, nausea and respiratory depression are well recognised.[49] Acquired pharmacodynamic tolerance to opioids, that is from changes in disposition or metabolism of the drug on repeat dosing, has been demonstrated in animals,[50] and involves changes to opioid and NMDA receptors. Neuronal excitotoxicity is induced, thus increasing doses are needed to achieve the same clinical effect. NMDA receptor antagonists such as ketamine may prevent and reverse tolerance, and thereby hyperalgesia. Alternative opioids, particularly methadone, may have inherent NMDA antagonism, thus rotation is a reasonable therapeutic option. Tolerance to methadone has been described.[51] It has also been demonstrated that individuals receiving methadone maintenance (for drug abuse) have lower pain thresholds than controls,[52] though this may be a reflection of non-pharmacological influences.

- *dependency*: physical dependency is a state of adaptation that is manifested by a withdrawal syndrome on abrupt cessation and rapid dose reduction. It is not addiction and is an expected consequence to the administration of certain medications including opioids, benzodiazepines and corticosteroids. For most persons a few weeks of regular opioid use creates physical dependency. It is less likely, and probably does not occur, if the administered drug resolves a particular symptom (pain, anxiety) than if the drug is used for recreational purposes. 'Pseudo-addiction' refers to the seeking of additional medication secondary to under-treatment of pain. Clinically this may be encountered when managing pain in terminally ill substance-misusing patients – in addition to the opioid maintenance dose, these patients require an adequate analgesic dose (*see* Box 4.1). Careful monitoring, urine testing and very firm rules prohibiting abuses (intentional misuse) of prescription and supply are necessary for these patients (*see* Chapter 12).
- *opioid withdrawal syndrome*: in palliative care practice, withdrawal may occur when switching from morphine to fentanyl, awaiting its onset of action, or if the opioid rotation dose is grossly underestimated. Only 25% of the opioid dose is required to prevent withdrawal symptoms. The autonomic discomfort and agitation of opioid withdrawal is unpleasant, self-limiting and not medically dangerous unless otherwise the patient is physically unwell.
- *addiction*: the fear of addiction from the archetypal 'dangerous drug', morphine, is common in the general community. Addiction refers to a psychological dependence on a drug, compulsive use, continued use in spite of harm, craving for the drug and loss of control over usage. There is little evidence of addiction initiated by medicinal use, particularly in cancer patients. Of nearly 12,000 patients given opioids only four developed post-hospitalisation addiction, a rate of 0.03%.[53] Of 10,000 burns patients prescribed opioids, 22

Box 4.1 Terminology of drug behaviours

- Misuse: incorrect or improper use
- Abuse: intentional misuse
- Tolerance: the same dose resulting in a lesser effect
- Dependency: physiological adaptation and withdrawal symptoms on cessation
- Pseudo-addiction: seeking of additional medication due to undertreatment of pain
- Addiction: psychological dependency, compulsive use, craving, continued use in spite of harm, loss of control over usage

became addicted and all these individuals had a past history of drug abuse.[54] In patients with chronic pain conditions prescribed maintenance opioids, the risk of iatrogenic addiction is low, less than a few per cent, though the studies are hard to interpret.[55] There is no doubt that prior substance abuse increases the risk of addiction. The drug is not the sole factor in drug addiction.

Opioids other than morphine

Codeine
Initially isolated from opium in 1832, codeine's active component is predominantly morphine. The breakdown to morphine by the cytochrome P450 enzyme 2D6, cannot occur in about 10% of the population, who lack this enzyme. This pathway is also blocked by SSRIs (except citalopram).

Fentanyl
A synthetic pure mu opioid agonist developed initially in the 1950s, fentanyl is 70–80 times more potent than morphine. Originally used as an anaesthetic agent, a transdermal slow-release preparation was produced in the 1970s. The advantages are of a predictable release of analgesia over 72 h. However, some patients psychologically appreciate the attention and interest shown in the process of administering medications on a more frequent basis. Fentanyl possesses less neurotoxicity than does morphine. In some countries an oral transmucosal formulation is available. 'Lacing' or dangerously augmenting illicit opioids with fentanyl has recently been reported.

Oxycodone
A semi-synthetic opioid which targets the kappa as well as the mu receptors, oxycodone has been in clinical use since 1917. Derived from thebaine, it is twice as potent as morphine. Fewer hallucinations than with morphine have been reported.[56] The rapid-acting oxycodone has proved very popular as a street drug of abuse.

Hydromorphone
An analogue of morphine, hydromorphone was first synthesised in 1921. It is 7.5 times more potent and perhaps has less neurotoxic adverse effects than does morphine.

Pethidine
Pethidine, first synthesised in 1939, should no longer be used in medicine. It has been shown to be devoid of analgesic effect (particularly the oral formulation). It provides relief because of its strong psychotomimetic (exhilaration and sedation) action.[57] Its action on the sphincter of Oddi is no less than that of other opioids. The major metabolite of pethidine, norpethidine, accumulates and is neurotoxic. Myoclonus, agitation and seizures may occur. Onoing use of parenteral pethidine is highly addictive and not recommended.

Buprenorphine

A semi-synthetic partial mu agonist, with delta and kappa activity, buprenorphine is safer in overdosage. Recently available as a transdermal preparation it is establishing a role in palliative care. Naloxone may be combined with buprenorphine to enhance its safety in a drug-abusing population.

Methadone

Primarily a mu agonist, methadone also has NMDA antagonist activity and inhibits the re-uptake of serotonin and noradrenaline in the spinal cord. First produced during World War II in Germany, it wasn't until post-war that the clinical usefulness of this compound was fully appreciated. Methadone is today stigmatised because of its use in substance abuse clinics. It is as effective an analgesic as morphine. Preferably it should be prescribed as split dosing for pain (in contrast to drug abuse). The advantages of methadone are that it is effective and cheap, however because of its long and individually variable half-life (15–120 h), toxicity is a significant risk, especially in the elderly. Conversion doses from morphine are difficult to estimate. It has (unproven) efficacy in neuropathic pain. It is less sedating than morphine and has less appeal for illicit users.

Diamorphine (heroin)

Diamorphine is an opioid with 6–7 times the potency of morphine. No substantial therapeutic differences to morphine have been demonstrated, in spite of clinicians' impressions that it is more effective.

Naloxone

An essential opioid antagonist in palliative care settings, naloxone also possesses, at very low dosage, analgesic augmentation properties when combined with morphine. Indeed if given in the absence of other opioids, naloxone has mild analgesic action.

Tramadol

Tramadol is a weak opioid analgesic but also facilitates the release of noradrenaline and serotonin in the descending inhibitory pain pathways of the spinal cord. Tramadol binding to the mu-opioid receptor is 6000 times weaker than that of morphine, therefore its analgesic action is likely to be predominantly monoamine related.[58] It is used as a step 2 option on the WHO analgesic ladder.[31] Its efficacy may be similar to codeine (it is a synthetic analogue of codeine). It may have efficacy in neuropathic pain,[12] though it is used widely as a general analgesic. Convulsions have been reported in those with a history of epilepsy, those on high dosage or those using it in combination with other psychotropics such as SSRIs and TCAs.[58] Sedation is rare. Abuse potential is very low, as are the risks of dependence and tolerance.[58] There has been very widespread use of this compound, and its safety appears well established. Drug interactions can occur with concomitant use of cytochrome P (CYP)3A4 inducers (e.g. carbamazapine), and serotonin enhancers (monoamine oxidase inhibitors (MAOIs)). Interactions with SSRIs may cause serotonin syndrome; however this appears to be rare in clinical practice. The molecular structure of tramadol is remarkably similar to that of the antidepressant venlafaxine, and there have been case reports of its anti-depressant activity.[59]

Non-opioid analgesics

Non-steroidal anti-inflammatory drugs (NSAIDs)

NSAIDs are particularly indicated for boney pain and do have some opioid-sparing activity. NSAIDs inhibit platelet aggregation. SSRIs affect platelet function, thus the combination may enhance the risk of gastrointestinal bleeding. Prostaglandins play a role in memory consolidation, and subjective cognitive impairments have been anecdotally reported with NSAIDs. These deficits are subtle and only recognised in a small minority. They are probably not of clinical significance.

Antidepressant medications

The use of antidepressant medications in a wide variety of chronic pain syndromes, including cancer and neuropathic pains, is usual clinical practice. Determining their actual effectiveness as co-analgesics is difficult. TCAs are effective for post-herpetic neuralgia.[60] The number needed to treat to achieve at least 50% pain relief compared to a placebo is 2.3.[60] Similar efficacy has been shown in diabetic neuropathy, atypical facial pain and post-stroke pain.[60] They do appear to have analgesic effect independently of their action on mood.[61] The median required dosage is lower than the usual dosage required to treat major depression, and the onset of action occurs faster (one to seven days).[61] That antidepressants are more effective for 'burning' pain than for 'shooting' pains has been dismissed.[61] The different TCAs do not exhibit different analgesic efficacies.[60] Amitriptyline is the most commonly used TCA, nortriptyline has the least adverse reactions and imipramine is the cheapest. There is no evidence that newer antidepressants are more effective co-analgesics. The number to treat to achieve 50% relief in neuropathic pain is 5.0 for paroxetine and 15.3 with fluoxetine. Mianserin is ineffective.[60] Opioid sparing has been demonstrated in cancer patients. The primary problem with the use of TCAs is their adverse effect profile.[12] Caution is required in those with cardiovascular histories, glaucoma, urinary retention and autonomic neuropathy. Particular sensitivity to the adverse effects of antidepressant medications is known to occur in pain patients. They may cause balance problems (a threefold increase in rate of falls) and cognitive impairment because of their anticholinergic effects. About one-third of medically ill patients have to withdraw from TCAs because of intoler-able adverse reactions.[62] Amitriptyline, the most toxic (even at low dosage), is metabolised to its active component, nortriptyline. Nortriptyline is a very much more tolerable drug and equipotent to amitriptyline in post-herpetic neuralgia. Very low dosage (e.g. 5 mg nocte) should be introduced and gently titrated upwards over several weeks to 25–50 mg nocte. The antidepressant range of nortriptyline is 50–100 mg. Serum drug levels of nortriptyline, but not the other dirtier TCAs, are accurate and can be useful in determining toxic doses (and therapeutic doses in depression treatment). Mirtazepine, with its sedating prop-erties, and venlafaxine, which is broad-spectrum in action, are increasingly used for depression and pain indications.

Putative mechanisms of action include direct action on monoamine transmitters enhancing inhibitory pathways, adenosinergic effects and antihistaminic effects. Low dosage regimes and rapid onset suggests the possibility of a direct analgesic action. Definitively diagnosing major depressive episodes in the presence of pain is difficult. Their usefulness in neuropathic pain may be accounted for by the effects on sleep. 'Improved sleep may be a huge bonus.'[60] No comparative trials of TCAs and an effective hypnotic have been published. The considerable therapeutic faith placed in TCAs as adjuvant analgesics may be an expression of our desperation in managing difficult pain. It is clinically convenient to offer another medication trial rather than admit therapeutic defeat in the face of such terrible torment.

Anticonvulsant medications

These may be used as co-analgesics in neuropathic pain. Gabapentin, the best-studied of the anticonvulsants for neuropathic pain, is effective at high dosage (3600 mg/day) in post-herpetic neuralgia and diabetic neuropathy.[63] In uncontrolled trials, positive effects on other neuropathic pain syndromes were demonstrated. Gabapentin is less effective than opioids in neuropathic pain.[11] Tolerability is good, though drowsiness may occur, particularly if dose escalation is rapid. Anticonvulsants can cause significant cognitive adverse reactions, predominantly a consequence of their sedative effects. At high dosage, ataxia and cognitive impairment (in the elderly) may be induced. Because of the need to slowly escalate the dosage, a therapeutic trial of up to 2 months is advisable. Gabapentin is now considered a first-line anticonvulsant medication in neuropathic pain. Carbamazepine, sodium valproate, phenytoin and lamotrigine have limited proven efficacy.

Ketamine

Burst subcutaneous (or oral) ketamine may be used as an analgesic for neuropathic and inflammatory pain, and to reset opioid receptors in high-dose opioid regimes. An NMDA receptor antagonist, ketamine, at subanaesthetic doses blocks the effects of the main excitatory transmitter in the CNS, glutamate. The phenomenon of opioid 'wind-up' or central sensitisation (rapid opioid escalation with diminishing responsiveness) may be arrested by pulses of ketamine. 'Wind-up' refers to the triad of allodynia, hyperalgesia and prolongation of the pain response (failing opioid responsiveness). The commonest adverse reactions of ketamine are psychiatric – vivid dreams/nightmares, dissociative sensations (such as feeling detached from one's body, misperceptions), dysphoria, visual hallucinations and, rarely, delirium. These adverse reactions are rare with the minute doses used for palliative care indications, and the warning that ketamine should be used with caution in those with a psychiatric history is probably overstated. Dose reduction and/or the introduction of as required midazolam (5 mg SC Stat) or haloperidol (2–5 mg PO/SC Stat) contain these adverse effects. Clozapine may be more effective than haloperidol at blunting the NMDA antagonist-induced psychosis in schizophrenic patients administered ketamine.[64] Amantadine or opioid rotation with methadone, both of which have NMDA antagonism, may be alternatives in those with fragile mental states and who are in need of addressing paradoxical pain syndromes.

Psychostimulants

Psychostimulants, because of their arousing action, can reverse opioid-induced sedation, thereby allowing an increase of opioid if necessary. Indirectly they enhance analgesia. Only at very high dose (100–300 mg amphetamine) are they liable to induce psychosis. A past history of psychosis is a relative contra-indication to their use. At methylphenidate doses of less than 1 mg/kg it is unlikely that psychiatric adverse reactions, including dependence, will result.

Benzodiazepines

The hypnotic qualities of benzodiazepines tend to fade after several weeks of regular use. They hasten the onset of sleep and prolong the phase of light sleep, hence increasing total sleep time. Non-benzodiazepine hypnotics such as zopiclone and zolpidem are preferred as these cause fewer changes in the sleep stages. They also act upon the GABA receptor, and their mechanism of action is similar to that of benzodiazepines. The differences may be related to dose and half-life of the respective compounds. Clonazepam, for its anticonvulsant properties, may be a tolerable option for neuropathic pain. In this instance, tolerance does not usually occur, and a stable dose should remain therapeutic.

References

1   Kingsley C. St Maura. AD304. *Poems*. London: Macmillan; 1872, p. 243.
2   Proust M. Cities of the Plain. *Remembrance of Things Past*. Vol. 7. (tr. CK Scott Moncrieff). London: Chatto & Windus: 1952, p. 199.
3   Merskey H. The definition of pain. *Eur J Psychiatry*. 1991; 6: 153–9.
4   Turk DC. The role of psychological factors in chronic pain. *Acta Anaesthesiol Scand*. 1999; 43: 885–8.
5   Fillingim RB. Sex, gender, and pain: women and men really are different. *Curr Rev Pain*. 2000; 4: 24–30.
6   Ferrell BA. Pain management. *Clin Geriatr Med*. 2000; 16: 853–74.
7   Farrar JT, Young JP Jr, La Mooreaux L *et al*. Clinical importance of changes in chronic pain intensity measured on an 11-point numerical rating scale. *Pain*. 2001; 94: 149–58.
8   Clark JP. Chronic pain prevalence and analgesic prescribing in a general medical population. *J Pain Symptom Manage*. 2002; 23: 131–7.
9   Portenoy RK and Lesage P. Management of cancer pain. *Lancet*. 1999; 353: 1695–700.
10 Glare P, Aggarwal G and Clark K. Ongoing controversies in the pharmacological management of cancer pain. *Int Med J*. 2004; 34: 45–9.
11 Eisenberg E, McNicol ED and Carr DB. Efficacy and safety of opioid agonists in the treatment of neuropathic pain of nonmalignant origin: systematic review and meta-analysis of randomized controlled trials. *JAMA*. 2005; 293: 3043–52.
12 Dworkin RH, Backonja M, Rowbotham MC et al. Advances in neuropathic pain. *Arch Neurol*. 2003; 60: 1524–34.
13 Blair MJ, Robinson RL, Katon W *et al*. Depression and pain co-morbidity: a literature review. *Arch Intern Med*. 2003; 163: 2433–5.
14 Aristotle. Quoted in: Fernandez E. *Anxiety, Depression and Anger in Pain*. Dallas: Advanced Psychological Resourcs; 2002.
15 McCracken LM and Iverson GL. Predicting complaints of impaired cognitive functioning in patients with chronic pain. *J Pain Symptom Manage*. 2001; 21: 392–6.

16 Spiegel D and Bloom JR. Pain in metastatic breast cancer. *Cancer.* 1993; 52: 341–5.

17 Padilla G, Ferrell B, Grant M *et al.* Defining the content domain of quality of life for cancer patients with pain. *Cancer Nursing.* 1990; 13: 108–15.

18 Okifugi A, Turk DC, Curran SL *et al.* Anger in chronic pain: investigations of anger targets and intensity. *J Psychosom Res.* 1999; 47: 1–12.

19 Merskey H. Pain and psychological medicine. In: Wall PD and Melzach R (eds). *Textbook of Pain* (4e). Edinburgh: Churchill Livingstone; 1999, pp. 929–49.

20 Beecher H. Pain in men wounded in battle. *Ann Surg.* 1946; 123: 96–105.

21 Engel GL. 'Psychogenic' pain and the pain-prone patient. *JAMA.* 1959; 26: 899–918.

22 Hackett TP and Bouckoms A. The pain patient: evaluation and treatment. In: Hackett TP and Cassem NH (eds). *Massachusetts General Hospital Handbook of General Hospital Psychiatry* (2e). Littleton: PSG Publishing Co; 1987, p. 43.

23 Saunders C. The philosophy of terminal care. In: Saunders C (ed). *The Management of Terminal Disease.* London: Edward Arnold; 1978.

24 Simon GE, van Korff M, Piccinelli M *et al.* An international study of the relationship between somatic complaints and depression. *N Engl J Med.* 1999; 341: 1329–35.

25 von Knorring L, Perris C, Eisemann M *et al.* Pain as a symptom in depressive disorders. II. Relationship to personality traits as assessed by means of KSP. *Pain.* 1983; 17: 377–84.

26 Breitbart W. Suicide in cancer patients. *Oncology.* 1987; 1: 49–53.

27 Moldofsky H. Sleep and pain. *Sleep Med Rev.* 2001; 5: 385–93.

28 Onen SH, Onen F, Courpron P *et al.* How pain and analgesics disturb sleep. *Clin J Pain.* 2005; 21: 422–31.

29 Merlin MD. *On the Trail of the Ancient Opium Poppy.* London: Associated University Press; 1984.

30 Dikotter F, Laamann L and Zhou X. *Narcotic Culture: a history of drugs in China.* Chicago: University of Chicago Press; 2004.

31 World Health Organization. *Cancer Pain Relief.* Geneva: WHO; 1986.

32 Moore P and Dimsdale JE. Opioids, sleep and cancer-related fatigue. *Med Hypotheses.* 2002; 58: 7782.

33 Morita T, Otani H, Tsanoda J *et al.* Successful palliation of hypoactive delirium due to multi-organ failure by oral methylphenidate. *Support Care Cancer.* 2000; 8: 134–7.

34 Lawler PG. The panorama of opioid-related cognitive dysfunction in patients with cancer: a critical literature appraisal. *Cancer.* 2002; 94: 1836–53.

35 Ersek M, Cherrier MM, Overman SS *et al.* The cognitive effects of opioids. *Pain Manag Nurs.* 2004; 5: 75–93.

36 Ashby MA, Martin P and Jackson KA. Opioid substitution to reduce adverse effects in cancer pain management. *Med J Aust.* 1999; 170: 454–5.

37 Raja SN, Haythornthwaite JA, Pappagallo M *et al.* Opioids versus antidepressants in postherpetic neuralgia: a randomised, placebo-controlled trial. *Neurology.* 2002; 59: 1015–21.

38 Fountain A. Visual hallucinations: a prevalence study among hospice inpatients. *Palliat Med.* 2001; 15: 19–25.

39 Vainio A, Ollila J, Matikanen E *et al.* Driving ability in cancer patients receiving long-term morphine analgesia. *Lancet.* 1995; 346: 667–70.

40 Bodkin JE, Zornberg GL, Lukas SE et al. Buprenorphine treatment of refractory depression. *J Clin Psychopharmacol.* 1994; 15: 49–57.

41 MacDonald M. *Mystical Bedlam: madness, anxiety, and healing in seventeenth-century England.* Cambridge: Cambridge University Press; 1981, p. 190.

42 Varga E, Sugerman A and Apter J. The effect of codeine on involutional and senile depression. *Ann NY Acad Sci*. 1982; 398: 103–5.

43 Kaiko RF, Wallenstein SL, Rogers AD *et al*. Analgesic and mood effects of heroin and morphine in cancer patients with postoperative pain. *N Engl J Med*. 1981; 304: 1501–6.

44 Romach MK, Sproule BA, Sellers EM *et al*. Long-term codeine use is associated with depressive symptoms. *J Clin Psychopharmacol*. 1999; 19: 373–6.

45 Martin WR. History and development of mixed opioid agonists, partial agonists and antagonists. *Br J Clin Pharm*. 1979; 7: 273S–279S.

46 Mercadante S, Ferrera P, Villari P *et al*. Hyperalgesia: an emerging iatrogenic syndrome. *J Pain Symptom Manage*. 2003; 26: 769–75.

47 Mao J, Sung B, Ji R-R *et al*. Neuronal apoptosis associated with morphine tolerance: evidence for an opioid-induced neurotoxic mechanism. *J Neurosci*. 2002; 22: 7650–61.

48 Bruera E and Kim HN. Cancer pain. *JAMA*. 2003; 290: 2476–9.

49 Fainsinger RL and Bruera E. Is this opioid analgesic intolerance? *J Pain Symptom Manage*. 1995; 10: 573–7.

50 Collett B-J. Opioid tolerance: the clinical perspective. *Br J Anaesth*. 1998; 81: 58–68.

51 Garrido MJ and Troconiz IF. Methadone: a review of its pharmacokinetic/ pharmacodynamic properties. *J Pharmacol Toxicol Methods*. 1999; 42: 61–6.

52 Weaver M and Scholl S. Abuse liability in opioid therapy for pain treatment in patients with an addictive history. *Clin J Pain*. 2002; 18(suppl): S61–9.

53 Porter J and Jick H. Addiction rare in patients treated with narcotics. *N Eng J Med*. 1980; 302: 123.

54 Perry S and Heidrich G. Management of pain during debridement: a survey of US burn units. *Pain*. 1982; 13: 267–80.

55 Littlejohn C, Baldacchino A and Bannister J. Chronic non-cancer pain and opioid dependence. *J R Soc Med*. 2004; 97: 62–5.

56 Maddocks I, Somogyi A, Abbott F *et al*. Attenuation of morphine-induced delirium in palliative care by substitution with infusion of oxycodone. *J Pain Symptom Manage*. 1996; 12: 182–9.

57 Olofsson CH, Ekblom A, Ekman-Ordeberg G *et al*. Lack of analgesic effect of systemically administered morphine or pethidine on labour pain. *Br J Obstet Gynaecol*. 1996; 103: 968–72.

58 Bamigbade TA and Langford RM. The clinical use of tramadol hydrochloride. *Pain Reviews*. 1998; 5: 155–82.

59 Markowitz JS and Patrick KS. Venlafaxine-tramadol similarities. *Med Hypotheses*. 1998; 51: 167–8.

60 McQuay HJ and Moore RA. Antidepressants and chronic pain. *BMJ*. 1997; 314: 763–4.

61 Max MB, Lynch SA, Muir J *et al*. Effects of desipramine, amitriptyline, and fluoxetine on pain in diabetic neuropathy. *N Engl J Med*. 1992; 326: 1250–6.

62 Popkin M, Callies A and Mackenzie T. The outcome of antidepressant use in the medically ill. *Arch Gen Psychiatry*. 1985; 42: 1160–3.

63 Mellegers MA, Furlan AD and Mailis A. Gabapentin for neuropathic pain: systematic review of controlled and uncontrolled literature. *Clin J Pain*. 2001; 17: 284–95.

64 Malhotra AK, Adler CM, Kennison SD *et al*. Clozapine blunts NMDA antagonist-induced psychosis: a study with ketamine. *Biol Psychiatry*. 1997; 42: 664–8.

Chapter 5

Other symptoms and the psyche

The brain and the mind effect and are affected by the systemic symptoms of advanced malignancy.

Pruritis

Pruritis (itch) is an unpleasant cutaneous sensation which provokes the desire to scratch.[1] Cough can be considered as a respiratory itch. Like pain it serves a protective function. It can be conceptualised as a type of pain. Released histamine and other pruritogens provoke the motor response of scratching. Itch is a common symptom in advanced malignancy. It may accompany cholestasis and uraemia. It frequently occurs in blood disorders and HIV/AIDS. Cytokines released by tumours may provoke itch, and peripheral nerve lesions may induce it. Local factors such as dry skin may contribute to pruritis, though central influences are important. Psychological and psychiatric influences are clinically relevant. Medications are more often the cause than the cure of itch. Generalised itch occurs in about 1% of those receiving oral opioids, and at considerably greater frequency in those on parenteral opioids.[2] This appears to be a central effect. Mu receptors mediate itch, and kappa receptors block itch. This adverse effect is usually self-limiting.

Topical treatments of itch – emollients, cooling, calamine, antihistamines, capsaicin – may be of only limited value. Systemic treatment with the older generation of antihistamines (e.g. promethazine) can result in over-sedation. Antidepressant medications, particularly doxepin (a crude but effective antihistamine-like tricyclic) and paroxetine, can be helpful for weeks to months, but efficacy tends to fade. Paroxetine, at low dosage, seems more effective than other SSRIs, for unknown reasons. Mirtazapine may have a role in managing itch, and opioid antagonists decrease scratching in cholestatic itch and severe uraemia. Corticosteroids are often empirically trialled. Pruritis is disturbing and distressing. If persistent, like pain, it tends to induce negative affect and cognitions.

Fatigue/asthenia

> If I had strength enough to hold a pen, I would write how easy and pleasant a thing it is to die.
>
> William Hunter (1718–1783)[3]

Fatigue is the commonest symptom experienced during the course of cancer, with prevalence estimates of greater than 70–80%. Often not volunteered, upon asking most cancer patients, as well as those with neurodegenerative disorders, complain of this debilitating symptom. The lay terms are tiredness or exhaustion. Fatigue is difficult to quantify. It is entirely a subjective symptom. It is not the same as muscle weakness, rather it is difficulty in the initiation, or sustaining, of voluntary activities.[4] The medical term asthenia includes fatigue, generalised weakness and mental fatigue. It refers to decreased capacity to maintain adequate performance (tiring easily), difficulties initiating activity, impaired concentration and memory, and emotional lability.[5] Poor concentration, forgetfulness, making slips of the tongue and being unable to find the correct word are typical subjective complaints of tired persons, yet on formal neuropsychological testing objective deficits are not usually confirmed.[6] With advancing disease, fatigue tends to progress to such an extent that it precludes independent functioning. The concept of 'vital exhaustion', initially used in cardiology,[7] aptly describes terminal fatigue.

Fatigue may be caused directly by the disease and indeed many patients attribute their fatigue to the cancer 'stealing' their energy. Damage to the nervous system results in profound fatigue, for the system is required to function at maximal capacity to cope with routine life tasks. Therapeutic 'poisons' such as chemotherapy and radiotherapy are potent causes of fatigue as are the array of medications with sedating side-effects. Tiredness is a sign of depression, a consequence of insomnia and a symptom of anxiety and worry. Clinically differentiating depression and fatigue is difficult.[8] The affective and cognitive symptoms differentiate them, but the physiological symptoms do not. There is overlap of symptoms between depression and fatigue. Neurasthenia is being reconsidered as a psychiatric syndrome for this reason. Fatigue is a cardinal symptom of anaemia and a clinical indicator of the need for blood transfusion. Physical disuse reinforces fatigue, and fatigue discourages activity. This vicious cycle not only undermines physical functioning, it erodes emotional wellbeing, and immobility encourages psychological regression (see Chapter 3).

Occasionally the cause may be reversed, but more commonly therapeutic endeavours fail. The important exception is if fatigue is symptomatic of depression. Some activity should be encouraged. Physiotherapy may be useful both functionally and psychologically. Corticosteroids may be trialled, and temporary respite can be achieved. Corticosteroids are perhaps best reserved for facilitating energy for an important occasion because of the risk of long-term adverse effects. Psychostimulants, modern day 'tonics', can be beneficial particularly in the earlier stages before the disease process has 'run down' the dopaminergic neurotransmitters.

Wretched as fatigue is, particularly to those who have led a physically active lifestyle, it does have protective and adaptive functions. By limiting the capacity to over-exertion and overwork, fatigue serves to biologically retain some reserve of energy. Psychologically, fatigue instructs the reluctant victim that physically they are not immortal, and that despite their hope to the contrary, death is approaching. Denial is challenged by this symptom. Appropriate dependency is enforced. A gradual withdrawal of attachment commences as the patient ceases to have the energy to participate in family and society events. A proclamation of surrender and a covenant of acceptance are provoked by vital fatigue.[9]

Nausea and vomiting

The prevalence of nausea in general population studies is about 10%.[10] Nausea is one of the most frequent and unpleasant symptoms associated with advanced malignancy. It is often the symptom of multiple pathological insults involving the pharynx and the gut, direct CNS exposure to toxic or pressure influences of malignancy, chemotherapy, radiotherapy, and opioid medication. Central structures involved in nausea, such as the chemoreceptor trigger zone and the 'vomiting centre' in the medulla, are vulnerable to emotional influence. In the last weeks of life, 80% of cancer patients require pharmacological interventions for nausea.

Derived from the Greek term for sea-sickness, nausea is 'a feeling of sickness with an inclination to vomit'. The term is not necessarily widely known in the general community, but the 'feeling of wanting to vomit' and similar terms are. Retching and vomiting may provide temporary relief from nausea. Nausea is often accompanied by autonomic arousal. Drowsiness is an associated symptom, and relief of nausea may enhance alertness. The malaise, dysphoria and apathy of motion sickness are known to us all. Anxiety is both a consequence of, and an aggravating influence on nausea.[10] It is under-appreciated that nausea may be a symptom of a major depressive episode, particularly in the elderly.[10]

Management of 'gut-related' nausea involves avoiding and minimising olfactory and food cues. Acupressure may assist. Most anti-emetic medications are psychoactive, exerting their actions on dopamine, histamine, serotonin and acetylcholine receptors. Adverse effects of these central acting medications are to be expected. Metoclopramide, the drug of choice for 'gut-related' nausea, can induce acute dystonic reactions, most commonly in young adults. Akathisia may occur with prolonged use. Metoclopramide is often not registered by clinicians as being a phenothiazine, and its potential to cause neurological adverse effects not considered. Domperidone has similar prokinetic action, but because it does not cross the bloodbrain barrier it does not cause neurological adverse effects. Levomepromazine is sedating and liable to induce postural hypotension and extrapyramidal adverse effects in the elderly and the frail. Anticholinergic and antimuscarinic medications such as these anti-emetics are prone to exacerbate cognitive difficulties.

Opioid-induced nausea, which occurs in 10–40% of patients at the commencement of opioid therapy, is most common with morphine and is generally relieved with central acting anti-emetics such as haloperidol (at dosages of less than 1–2 mg). Prophylactic anti-emetics are not required, but should be easily accessed if needed. Semi-synthetic opioids are less inclined to induce nausea. For most this nausea is a self-limiting symptom, and within weeks tolerance develops.

Motion-induced nausea, a conflict between visual and vestibular sensors, can worsen rapidly (the avalanche syndrome) and be mercifully relieved by vomiting. Females suffering gynaecological cancers are at particular risk for this variant of nausea. This type of nausea is the most vulnerable to psychological influences, particularly expectation. Motion sickness can reduce pain sensitivity in a way analogous to stress-induced analgesia.[11] In addressing motion sickness, adequate analgesia is necessary and this may need to be administered parenterally until control is regained. Attending to the mismatch between visual and vestibular information is difficult, if not impossible, as the movement inducing the nausea is commonly as simple as altering body posture in bed. Cyclizine and hyoscine, usual medications of early choice for motion sickness, may be sedating. Because levomepromazine hits multiple receptors it can be effective. Adventure sportsmen, at high risk for motion sickness, tend to opt for the phenothiazine antihistamine drug promethazine. Interestingly after about 5 days at sea, sea sickness usually resolves spontaneously. This is not necessarily so for space sickness nor for the nausea of advanced disease. For several days after return to land, sea sickness may resurge (*mal de débarquement*). It is therefore clinically sensible to be patient and cautious, for successful relief of motion sickness may take several days to 'bed-down'. Habituation does not appear to occur in cancer-related nausea, unlike sea sickness. Fear and expectation seem more potent behavioural influences than desensitisation. Acupuncture and diet have no scientific support as interventions.[12] Gastric stasis can be produced by motion sickness, resulting in secondary 'gut-related' nausea and poor oral absorption of anti-emetics.[12]

At least one-third of nauseous patients require multiple anti-emetics. The pharmacology of treating this symptom can easily become complicated. The most effective of the anti-emetics is a corticosteroid,[13] but this exposes the patient to many potential adverse effects, especially if long-term use is necessary. Serotonin ($5HT_3$) antagonists such as ondansetron are usually ineffective, but not invariably so. Benzodiazepines and phenytoin can be effective.[12] Neurokinin 1 receptor antagonists may find a role in palliative medicine. Managing nausea is 'trial and error' pharmacotherapy.

Anticipatory nausea and vomiting is triggered by *in vivo* exposure to certain stimuli associated with the administration of chemotherapy. It is a conditioned response and is amenable to behavioural intervention. Undoubtedly a concerning problem in oncological practice, it is of lesser relevance in palliative care.

Anorexia and cachexia

> When thou doste feele creepinge tyme at thye gate, these fooleries will please thee lesse; I am paste my relishe for such matters: thou seest my bodilie meate doth not suit me well; I have eaten but one ill tasted cake since yesternighte.
>
> Queen Elizabeth I (1533–1603)[14]

Diminishing and changing taste sensation and appetite occur in most advanced cancer patients. The causes are multiple. It is important to exclude depression as a cause, for this is potentially treatable. Attention to oral hygiene, small attractive meals and appetite stimulants may be of benefit. High-calorie food supplements are frequently advised but are of limited value aside from their psychological punch (often for the relative rather than the patient). Corticosteroids, prokinetic agents and psychostimulants may be trialled, though their value is questionable. Paradoxically, psychostimulants in the medically ill enhance appetite, whereas in the healthy they may be used and abused in order to lose weight. Progestogens are favoured by some, though evidence of efficacy is lacking. A small amount of alcohol prior to a meal may encourage appetite. Patients in the advanced stages of cancer often use the phrase 'fed-up' to describe this state, as if to suggest their appetite is satiated and they have no physiological need of food (despite the wasting). This contrasts sharply with the high rate of hospitalised elderly with critical non-malignant illnesses who are malnourished and interested in food.

The metabolic mechanism of the progressive wasting in advanced cancer and AIDS patients is uncertain. Cytokines are implicated. Cachexia is not starvation, and parenteral feeding does not reverse it. There are no effective treatments, though many approaches are usually tried. It is distressing for the patient to experience the withering loss of their familiar body shape and their strength. The changing body image challenges self-esteem (*see* Chapter 3). Sharing food with others is a social event, an important opportunity for communication, and a mode of expressing personal and cultural customs. Preparing food has immense communication and caring value. These losses for the cachexic patient may marginalise them, alienate them from their culture and deprive them of that precious time with others. Cachexia advertises sickness and dying.

Dyspnoea

Advanced cancer is commonly associated with dyspnoea, affecting perhaps 50%. Fears of inability to breathe and suffocation are difficult to manage, for respiratory failure is a feature of many terminal illnesses. It is a particular feature of advanced motor neurone disease. Difficulties acquiring sufficient oxygen activate the Hering–Breuer reflex, resulting in rapid, shallow breathing. This is a physiological attempt to compensate. However it also provokes anxiety, which, if intense, will undermine breathing efficiency. Posture, relaxation exercises, distraction and a fan blowing cool air at the face may be of benefit in the early stages. By consciously focusing on slowing the breathing rate, thereby enhancing its efficiency, the anxiety of respiratory distress may be eased. Hypoxia may be eased by oxygen therapy, at least transiently, provided the patient is not tolerant to carbon dioxide respiratory drive. Psychological dependency on oxygen, and the awkward and potentially dangerous equipment necessary, are important issues needing to be considered prior to providing this treatment. Sleep is invariably disrupted by dyspnoea, for both physiological and psychological reasons. In sleep, respiratory performance falls and these patients can't afford for this to occur. It is slightly more common to die at night, and fears of not awakening are not surprising. This may be of comfort to some, but disturbing to those not as yet accepting. Opioids and benzodiazepines can be most helpful in the advanced stages of respiratory failure, by slowing rate and relieving anxiety. Respiratory depression and hypercapnia are relative considerations only. Pain tends to protect against opioid-induced respiratory depression, and by this stage of illness most have current exposure to opioid medication. Symptom relief is a more pressing concern. The mechanism of opioids in this clinical situation is uncertain. Probably opioids function predominantly as anxiolytics. They may reduce the sensitivity of the 'respiratory centre' to oxygen and carbon dioxide stimulation, thereby slowing respiratory rate. Oral benzodiazepines, in contrast to parenteral benzodiazepine in the naive patient, have not been shown to adversely affect respiratory function. Chlorpromazine and buspirone have also been used for these symptoms.

Air hunger invokes distress. It may be that the attending relatives are more distraught by this than the patient. It is unlikely that sufficient consciousness is retained for a patient to be disturbed by Cheyne Stokes respiration and the 'death rattle'. It is important to note that while it is preferable to introduce anticholinergic medications early for retained salivation in those too weak to expectorate, such agents are potent precipitators of delirium. Glycopyrronium has a less delirogenic potential. Helpless relatives require reassurance and education regarding these disturbing physiological events. Profound and acute dyspnoea may be an indication for terminal sedation (*see* Chapter 8).

References

1   Haffenreffer S (1660). From: Rothman S. Physiology of itching. *Physiol Rev*. 1941; 21: 357–81.
2   Twycross R, Greaves MW, Handwerker H *et al*. Itch: scratching more than the surface. *Q J Med*. 2003; 96: 7–26.
3   Hunter J. Quoted by SR Gloyne. *John Hunter*. Edinburgh: E & S Livingstone; 1950, p. 88
4   Chaudhuri A and Behan PO. Fatigue in neurological disorders. *Lancet*. 2004; 363: 978–88.
5   Watanabe S and Bruera E. Anorexia and cachexia, asthenia and lethargy. In: Cherny NI and Foley KM (eds). Pain and palliative care. *Hematol Oncol Clin North Am*. 1996; 10: 189–206.
6   Moss-Morris R, Petrie K, Large R *et al*. Neuropsychological deficits in chronic fatigue syndrome: artefact or reality? *J Neurol Neurosurg Psychiatry*. 1996; 60: 474–7.
7   Appels A and Mulder P. Excess fatigue as a precurser of myocardial infarction. *Eur Heart J*. 1988; 9: 758–64.
8   Reuter K and Harter M. The concepts of fatigue and depression in cancer. *Eur J Cancer Care*. 2004; 13: 127–34.
9   Nunez Olarte JM and Dickerson ED. Asthenia: is it more than a symptom (editorial). *Prog Pall Care*. 2000; 8: 126–7.
10 Haug TT, Mykletun A and Dahl AA. The prevalence of nausea in the community: psychological, social and somatic factors. *Gen Hosp Psychiatry*. 2002; 24: 81–6.
11 Drummond PD. Suppression of pain and the R2 component of the blink reflex during optokinetic stimulation. *Cephalalgia*. 2004; 24: 44–51.
12 Golding JF and Gresty MA. Motion sickness. *Curr Opin Neurol*. 2005; 18: 29–34.
13 Glare P, Pereira G, Kristjanson LJ *et al*. Systematic review of the efficacy of antiemetics in the treatment of nausea in patients with far-reaching cancer: a review. *Support Care Cancer*. 2004; 12: 432–40.
14 Harington J. *The Letters and Epigrams of Sir John Harington: together with the Prayse of Private Life*. McClure NE (ed). Philadelphia: University of Pennsylvania Press; 1930, p. 97.

Chapter 6

Depression

My body is sick but my mind is worse, engrossed in gazing endlessly upon its suffering.

Ovid (43 BC–17 AD)[1]

The word 'depression' has changed its meaning over recent decades. In colloquial use it means sadness. The older term, 'melancholia', is an awkward term and unlikely to assume common use. Clinical depression or major depressive disorder (MDD) is the medical term used to refer to the disease 'depression'. While a common disorder in the general community, and not surprisingly more prevalent in the sick, depression has assumed over recent decades greater familiarity. It is generally accepted that depression is under-recognised and undertreated in the terminally ill, more so in non-malignant forms of terminal illness.[2] Increasing public and professional knowledge about the illness and tolerable medication options however risk over-diagnosis and over-treatment of this disorder in the general community.

Depression is not the inevitable consequence of misfortune or severe illness. It is a serious and manageable disorder that needs to be recognised and treated. Clinical depression is distressing and emotionally painful. It lowers the pain threshold, it may reduce survival in cancer patients by interfering with treatment compliance and immunological parameters, it precipitates early admissions to palliative care facilities for it reduces the ability to self-care, and suicide is a possible consequence of the illness. In addition to the immense suffering associated with depression, it can impair cognition and distort decision-making ability. Depression erodes the quality of remaining life. Major depression is treatable. In the general population the success of combined antidepressant and psychotherapy is 85%.[3] While likely to be more difficult to treat in a physically unwell population, depression clearly warrants considerable attention as a symptom and syndrome in the dying.

The relationship between cancer and depression may be bidirectional. Depression can be an early or occult symptom of a malignancy, and is a common complication of cancer. Studies of mood and stress (particularly social support) adversely influencing immune status and increasing cancer risk are conflicting, but appealing.[4,5]

Sadness and grief

Grief is itself a med'cine.

William Cowper (1731–1800)[6]

Sadness is the normal response to loss. Grief is the psychological process initiated by the death of a loved and attached person. Sadness, tearfulness, insomnia, and haunting reminiscences about the deceased are typical symptoms. Not infrequently, the bereaved may experience fleeting auditory and visual pseudohallucinations of the deceased and perhaps a sense of presence. Waves of distress, the pangs of sadness, often cued by reminders and reminiscences, characterise grieving. In the intervening periods normal functioning occurs. Yearnings for the lost one trouble the grieving. Over time, the distress, sad mood and negative cognitions fade in intensity and frequency. Culture and sex are important determinants as to how grief is expressed. Sadness is not pathological. The disruption to the flow of life is transient. Despite the emotional pain of grief, it demands of the individual psychological creativity in order to 'replace' the loss with 'live' memories of the deceased. Intrapsychically, the lost person, if significant, is able to be forever recalled. Our losses are never irretrievably forgotten. Grief is never fully resolved. Life may be a procession of losses, however these vicissitudes of life serve to entice psychological growth, maturity and wisdom.

Anticipatory grief refers to the psychological work of the dying emotionally and cognitively preparing for loss of life. Most find this difficult. As symptom burden increases, and fate becomes clearer, this may serve to encourage this unenviable task. Gentle reminders, even confrontation, may be helpful, though some can't or won't prepare for death and die fighting the reality of nature. The offering of endless, increasingly futile, oncology treatment options or an unflinching faith in alternative medicine may hamper this process. Not only does good preparation appear to ease some of the anxieties for the dying, it provides the loved ones opportunities to embark, with initial assistance, on their journey of grief. We live in a death-denying and death-defying society. Comfort in managing grief is an essential skill for all who work in palliative care. Therapeutic moments to address grief issues occur in the shower, changing dressings, chatting about life experiences or tidying up the room. The stilted and artificial situation of an office-based session of grief counselling is rarely ideal.

Complicated grief

Severe and prolonged grief may be indicative of co-morbid depression, substance abuse or other compounding psychiatric illness. Sudden, unexpected losses, particularly if the circumstances are traumatic and/or the attachment is uncertain or ambivalent, are risk factors for pathological grief reactions. Pre-existing psychiatric illness is likely to contaminate normal grief. If the tincture of time and support is not reshaping grief after several months, consideration of a co-existent depression should be made. Grief is a dynamic process, if it gets stuck or complicated, more expert psychotherapy and pharmacotherapy is indicated.

Diagnosing depression

> A cankered soul macerated with cares and discontents.
>
> Robert Burton (1577–1640)[7]

The symptoms of depression are affective, cognitive and somatic. Depression is best conceptualised as a spectrum disorder, the symptoms ranging from mild to very severe. As affect darkens, physical symptoms increasingly accompany and cognitions blacken. The differentiation between reactive and endogenous mood disorder is not particularly helpful. Negative life events may play a role precipitating depression, however this is somewhat uncertain. They are probably not more frequent than positive events precipitating a deterioration of mood. The changing circumstances force adaptation, and it may be this that unsettles mood equilibrium. The cause of depressive disorder is unknown. The inward turning of anger (the psychoanalytic model), pervasive negative thinking (Beck's cognitive model), learned helplessness (a behavioural model) and depression as a psychomotor disorder are useful theoretical concepts.[8] The catecholamine theory implicates biological changes, at least in severe depression. In cancer patients cytokines may play a role.[9] Mild depression may be a purely cognitive disruption, but with severity biology becomes progressively more relevant. There is a 'grey' zone along the spectrum where psychological and psychophysiological depressions merge. Clinical depression is a misery of mood. The sufferer pervasively feels low spirited, negative, pessimistic, lacking of enjoyment, incapable of pleasure, ruminative and worthless. Every moment the sufferer feels gloomy, sometimes (often early morning) more than at other times. Sadness is a frequent symptom, though not all acknowledge sadness. By diagnostic definition depressive symptoms need to persist for at least two weeks before being considered a disorder. It is not sensible clinical practice to diagnose depression on a single occasion. Reviewing on another occasion, perhaps the following day, provides a gauge of psychological reactivity and assists in differentiating major depression and sadness. Anhedonia and loss of interest in others, and in life, are prominent features. The patient becomes immersed in their own grim space. They 'hibernate' away from social contact. The future as perceived by the patient is beyond appreciation, for the present is so unbearable. Humour may not be lost, for much humour is indeed 'black'. The examiner may be 'touched' by the patient's sense of utter helplessness, this being a useful intuitive diagnostic indicator for experienced practitioners. Thoughts become muddy and sticky, self-centred and preoccupied with bleakness. Requesting euthanasia or accepting very high-risk treatment interventions may be indicative of this objectionable existence. Negativistic and nihilistic ideations and delusions may occur in severe depressive states. The pain of the emotions and thoughts of depressive disorder is so profound that self-destruction may emerge for the sufferer as a relieving and respectable option. The lifetime risk of attempted suicide of those suffering major depression is 25–50%. Intriguingly in Cotard's syndrome, a rare and severe psychotic depression, mood can paradoxically appear jovial despite the patient believing they 'no longer (deserve to) exist'. Life, to their great relief, has ended. A similar paradoxical affect may be observed in those patients who have formulated a definite plan to end their life, and in those physically recuperating following a suicide attempt. This seemingly improved mental status tends to persist only a few days before the misery resurfaces. Direct questioning of suicidal ideation and plans is essential, yet is by no means a guarantee of intent. In many ways, such intrusive interrogation is similar to a thorough physical examination. The patient is assured that their symptoms are being properly assessed.

Acquiring a history, a narrative, is an under-rated task in modern clinical medicine. It is the most valid assessment strategy. Information concerning the evolution of symptoms, past history and family history of affective disorder, substance use and medications is crucial. Obtaining corroborative information

Table 6.1 Major depressive disorder/dysthymia

Major depressive disorder	Dysthymic disorder
Symptom present >2 weeks	Symptom present >2 years
Depressed mood	Depressed mood
Insomnia (early morning awakening)	Insomnia (initial)/hypersomnia
Fatigue	Fatigue
Poor concentration/decision making	Poor concentration/decision making
Anhedonia/loss of interest	
Weight loss (>5%)	
Psychomotor retardation/agitation	
Worthlessness/guilt	
Suicidal ideation	Low self-esteem
	Hopelessness
Antidepressant medication responsive	

from important others (including attending health professionals) always assists, and in the frail terminally ill may be the only available option. The recognition of only 40% of depressions in cancer patients in the 1980s,[10] a reflection of similar difficulties in the general community, may have improved over recent decades. The reluctance of patients to disclose distress, for they assume that nothing could be done to alleviate it, or they don't wish to seem ungrateful, is undoubtedly a barrier hindering diagnosis.[11] The frank avoidance of medical staff asking about emotions (for fear of causing harm or being personally affected) and their distancing from the patient by presuming that the patient's emotional status is appropriate to their situation, by strategies such as premature reassurance or a change of topic, reduces the prospect of a psychiatric diagnosis.[11] A more recently acquired distancing strategy is that of a tearful patient being promptly prescribed antidepressant medication and dismissed.

The criteria-based signs and symptoms of MDD (*see* Table 6.1, DSM IV) are not so applicable to the medically ill. The core affective symptoms are depressed mood and anhedonia. The somatic symptoms such as insomnia, anorexia, cachexia, fatigue and motor retardation are less diagnostically discriminative in

---

Box 6.1 Affective and cognitive symptoms of major depression

- Dysphoric/depressed mood and affect
- Anhedonia
- Loss of interest/apathy
- Poor concentration/attention/memory
- Slowed/sluggish thoughts
- Pessimism/negativity
- Worthlessness/feeling a burden on others
- Excessive guilt
- Helplessness
- Hopelessness
- Suicidal ideation

the physically ill. The diagnosis in cancer patients rests upon the presence of affective and cognitive, rather than somatic, symptoms (*see* Box 6.1). The patient may be tearful, withdrawn, isolative, irritable and dismissive, and rejecting of attempts at establishing any human contact. And they may also be in pain. In the medically ill, the severity of the depression is not directly correlated with physical severity. About 10% of depressive illness has reverse or negative symptoms, such as overeating and hypersomnia. This hibernatory-type presentation is frequently missed. Age and sex influence the presentation of depressive symptoms. Behaviourally disruptive young children, withdrawn and irritable adolescents, anxious young women, aggressive men and cognitively slowed elderly portray the vast and varied pattern of affective disorders. Depression is by no means necessarily an easy diagnosis. The most widely used self-report measure of depression is the Hospital Anxiety and Depression Scale (HADS), which is a relatively easily administered tool. The Beck Depression Scale and many other scales tend to lose reliability in the presence of co-existent physical illness. These instruments are certainly indices of general distress, and are dependent upon the ability of the patient to respond to the questioning, but lack specificity for diagnosing MDD. They are useful research tools, but of limited assistance to the clinician. Not surprisingly Cochinov has shown that a single-item interview that asks 'are you depressed' is diagnostically of greater validity (and should be a routine admission question anyway).[12] Lloyd-Williams and co-workers suggested that this question is culturally specific and does not have the perfect sensitivity and specificity in the UK that it does in North America.[13] But by adapting the actual word to the society in which one works, Cochinov's question remains a robust and clinically very useful screening and diagnostic tool for MDD. 'Miserable', 'black', and 'low' tend to achieve similarly clinically valid responses. Co-opting the attention and co-operation of patients to complete assessment tools is usually only acceptable and feasible in those with mild to moderate disorder. In severe depression, the inability to perform such requests may be diagnostically relevant. However, of greatest significance to the clinician is the unproven relationship between these diagnostic tests and treatment responsiveness. Being able to anticipate medication-responsive depression is fundamentally what needs to be determined.

Prevalence

Depend upon it, Sir, when a man knows he is to be hanged in a fortnight, it concentrates his mind wonderfully.
Samuel Johnson (1709–1784)[14]

The current (1 month) prevalence of major depression in national epidemiological studies in the US, UK and Australasia is 3–5%.[15] Depression is commoner in women. Unipolar major depression in 1990 was the leading global cause of life-years lived with disability, and the fourth leading cause of disease burden. About one-quarter to one-third of medical inpatients and outpatients have some symptoms of depression, though generally these are milder than the symptoms encouraging presentation at a mental health service. The depression is severe in 4–18%, often in the more severely ill. Depression may precede the physical illness, more commonly it follows it.

A systematic review of the prevalence of depression in patients with advanced cancer and amongst mixed hospice populations in 2002 commented on the poor quality of available research.[16] Prevalence ranges from 1% to 50% depending upon methodological issues such as diagnostic criteria, method of diagnosis, the threshold of diagnosis and the incorporation or not of minor (adjustment, dysthymic) states.[17] From the clinician's perspective, relevant information required is whether or not antidepressant medications should be trialled. If affective symptoms are to the right of centre of the spectrum, then medication is likely to be appropriate. Minor depressions are unlikely to benefit from antidepressant medication. The HADS gave a median prevalence of 'definite depression' of 29%.[16] Using psychiatric interviews, the prevalence ranged from 5% to 26%, with a median of 15%.[17] 'Depression' frequently ranks in the 'top ten' symptoms in a hospice checklist, and the probability is that a proportion of cases are missed. Using stringent diagnostic criteria 5–15% of cancer patients meet criteria for MDD.[12] These patients require medication as a component of the management. A further 10–15% present with less severe 'subthreshold' depression, and at least 25% of advanced cancer patients present with a significant degree of dysphoria.[17,18] It is important to acknowledge that despite some uncertainties regarding exact prevalence, the vast majority of individuals with cancer do not develop clinical depression.

The separation of early- and late-stage cancer populations significantly influences prevalence figures. The stage or phase of the malignant illness is relevant. The major stress points during cancer are diagnosis, relapse, the introduction or removal of therapies and the moving from the curative to palliative phase. These periods are distressing, and potentially depressogenic. However so too may be the completion of a treatment modality, the consequential 'abandonment' by these providers, and the anxious awaiting of the feared relapse. The expected peak risk periods are early in the disease course, and late. There is an accumulation in the advanced phase of disease- and treatment-related burdens such as cytokine activity, physical frailty, chemotherapy side-effects, corticosteroid administration, pain and anticipatory grief. Much data suggest that depression is commoner in the later stages of illness, with prevalence rates of 13–26%.[18] However in the terminal phase, depression may be less frequent, even unusual. Conill surveyed by symptom questionnaire their subjects on two occasions, the second within 7 days of death, and noted a fall in the rate of depression from 53% to 39%.[19] Coyle retrospectively reviewed the files of 90 patients within 4 weeks of death by cancer, and noted that at 4 weeks 8% volunteered complaints of depression, and that this fell to 4% at one week.[20] Using DSM III criteria, a rate of MDD of only 3.2% was determined in 93 incurable and terminally ill patients, in a palliative care unit, who died within 6 months of admission.[21] Including disorders in which depressive affect plays a prominent part (MDD, adjustment disorders with depressed mood, minor depression), these authors observed only a 10% prevalence. Excluding the patients with cognitive impairment resulted in an overall prevalence of MDD of 6%.[21] As death approaches perhaps the rate of clinical depression actually falls, though not necessarily the rate of minor depression (or sadness). Depressive disorder is only rarely encountered in the dying, yet is common in the early and later phases of the cancer journey. Death on the horizon may be therapeutic for mood. Whether the mechanism for this is psychological or physiological, or both, is speculative. From an evolutionary perspective, depression is adaptive in situations where continued effort will result in either danger or loss of resources. Depressive symptoms inhibit challenging behaviours and de-escalate the conflict. Fighting for life becomes a futile effort and the 'need' to be depressed evaporates.[22] When there is no perceived or actual future, time is compressed to the immediate. Survival for the moment is the over-riding occupation.

The prevalence of depression in cancer patients has been lower during the last two decades than previously.[23] The speculative reasons for this are many, and the finding is not convincing as yet.

Risk factors

The aetiology of depressive illness is unknown. There are known factors which seem to be of relevance. There are minor genetic vulnerability factors, and psychological and physical stressors (*see* Box 6.2). That individuals become clinically depressed in response to changeable life events is not scientifically well established. The buffering effects of social support are difficult to prove. Contrary to risk factors for depression in the general population, depression of those with cancer may not be more prevalent in women and the aged. Depression is three times more prevalent among North American cancer patients who did not acknowledge their prognosis,[24] but this could be a consequence of the depression rather than a cause, for all would have been informed at some stage. In an Indian study the reverse trend has been described.[25] Particular diseases and medications are known to enhance risk. Depression can be a direct consequence of antineoplastic therapy. Among cancer patients the highest prevalence rates are exhibited in those patients with pancreatic, oropharyngeal and (early) breast cancers. Poorly controlled pain and increasing disease symptoms are associated with more severe depressions. The factors lowering resilience to depression

---

Box 6.2   Risk factors for major depression

- Genetic (family history of affective disorder, alcoholism)
- Past personal history
- Advanced age
- Advanced disease
- Oropharyngeal/pancreatic/(early) breast cancer
- Physical immobility/dependency
- Poorly controlled pain
- Social isolation/few social supports
- Alcohol
- Concurrent severe medical illness
- Medications:
  – corticosteroids
  – anabolic steroids
  – chemotherapy (vincristine, vinblastine, procabazine, interferons)
  – beta-blockers (propranolol)
  – ? benzodiazepines

---

cannot always be clinically identified. Depressive disorder is the final common pathway of internal and/or external disruption to the nervous system. Neuro-transmitter derangements do occur, but may be 'downstream' effects. What initiates this cascade of self-punitive biological events remains speculative. The popular explanation that depression is a deficit of nerve chemicals is convenient rather than convincing.

Differential diagnosis

The overwhelming sadness of the predicament of many terminally ill, projected onto the clinician, and the ill-informed carer's viewpoint 'that anyone in such circumstances would be depressed' may entice a relaxation of diagnostic rigour. Grief reactions are associated with undulations of mood and depression with a prostration of mood. Denial and manic defences, superficially protective to the sufferer, may dissuade the interviewer of the intensity of underlying distress. Adjustment disorder with depressed mood is a vague and impractical diag-nosis. Chronic dysthymia, predating the cancer, may encourage the clinician to formulate a depression diagnosis. Clinically differentiating 'major' and 'minor' depression is arbitrary at best. Uncharacteristic anxiety, particularly night-time panic attacks, may represent depression rather than an anxiety disorder. 'I can often find no proper differences between the sadness and the anxiety of the melancholic' wrote Lewis in 1934.[26] Major depressive disorder 'without mood symptoms', or a masked depression, is a recognised, though not fashionable, clinical state. Severe dysphoria tends not to be able to be hidden all the time, and the relative's history is often diagnostically pertinent. Differentiating mood and fatigue in the physically frail is difficult. The will to achieve a task is retained in the fatigued, though they don't possess the energy to accomplish the goal. 'I want to, but I can't' is different from 'I don't want to, and I won't'. 'Vital exhaustion' is that state of extreme physical, and indeed mental, fatigue caused by actual or impending physical ill-health.[27] Originally described as a precursor symptom to myocardial infarction, terminal malignancy eventually creates a similar state.

Sedative medications can induce depressed and unresponsive affect. Deterior-ating renal and hepatic functioning may induce toxicity of these and other previously tolerated medications. The psychomotor retardation of drug-induced parkinsonism mimics depression. Hypoactive delirium is easily misdiagnosed for MDD. Torporosed patients appear affectively flat and unreactive. The vague mentation consequent upon the cognitive inattention of AIDS and paraneo-plastic syndromes may seem affective, as may the gentle cognitive withdrawal of the dying as interest in the present is sacrificed and remaining energy focused on important interpersonal relationships. Nausea is an occasional depressive symptom, particularly in the elderly, and despondency associated with nausea is invariable.

The most challenging clinical dilemma is that of determining whether depressive disease is influencing those who have made a decision to decline active treatment when all medical hope is not lost. 'Giving up' in the face of insurmountable illness induces great concern, even anger, in relatives. It may be a depressive symptom. Alternatively it may be a sensible and responsible decision based on the reality of the clinical situation. If so, it tends to be 'affect neutral' and neither patient nor family wears the gloom or doom of depressed persons.

A rational and analytical account of the decision-making is provided, and rather than being hopeless, the patient has plans and expectations for the next and terminal phase of their illness. The 'giving up–given up' concept,[28] 'learned helplessness', abulia and apathy are distinctly different from the constructive and creative 'giving up'. Resignation in advanced malignancy is not pathological if it is based on a realistic appraisal of the future.

Demoralisation is a concept, recently championed by Kissane,[29] of particular relevance to palliative care patients. Demoralisation is a form of existential despair. The demoralised patient expresses non-specific dysphoria, such as distress, irritability, guilt or regret, and a growing sense of disheartenment. Loss of purpose and meaning can lead to helplessness, hopelessness, worthlessness and an impatient desire to die or hasten death.[29] Clinicians can perceive the demoralised to be contemplating 'rational' suicide. Up to 8% experience severe demoralisation which interferes with competency to make informed and autonomous choice, and may co-exist with or be a harbinger of clinical depression. Change in morale spans a spectrum of mental attitudes from disheartenment (mild loss of confidence), through despondency (starting to give up) and despair (losing hope) to demoralisation (having given up). Historical terms such as spiritual torpor, mopishness and acedia describe similar states of pointlessness and a non-caring attitude to living. The philosopher Kierkegaard describing the greatest despair of all stated: 'when death is the greatest danger, we hope for life; but when we learn to know even greater danger, we hope for death. When the danger is so great that death becomes the hope, then despair is the hopelessness of not even being able to die'.[30] Clinically it is possible to differentiate demoralisation and depression.[31] Demoralised patients, while feeling hopeless about their future, feel immediately content with their present. The core features of depression are anhedonia, the loss of both anticipatory and consummatory pleasure, and the loss of interest in life's activities. The demoralised feel no anticipatory pleasure, and are trapped and helpless. Still interactive with their environment, they are unable to conceive an escape from their distress except by death.[29] Whether demoralisation is a form of 'subthreshold' depression, an adjustment disorder, a form of reactive dysthymia, or a separate diagnosis is uncertain. Psychotherapeutic and social interventions of a supportive, empathic and reality-focused style may be of benefit rediscovering a meaning for the remainder of life.

Depression, suicide and desire to hasten death

Depression is a factor in at least 50% of all suicides. More women than men attempt suicide but because of choice of method, men are more likely to succeed. The peak incidences of completed suicide in the general population occur during adolescence and, for males, elderly age. The frequency of suicide in the cancer population is higher than in the general population,[32] with the highest risk in the months after diagnosis.[33] The risk decreases with survival time and is very low in the terminal phase.[34] Depression, uncontrolled pain, loss of control (helplessness) and advanced disease (exhaustion) are considered indicators of vulnerability to suicide in cancer patients.[18,35] Examination of coroner's files on suicides in elderly males showed that 20% had cancer identified at autopsy or had undergone treatment for cancer in the last year.[36] Of particular pertinence to the chronically physically ill, and not incorporated in suicide statistics, is neglect of personal care, non-compliance and inattention to the necessary care required by the disease. This carelessness may result in premature death. Depression and hopelessness are independent risk factors for suicide. At high levels of depression, the association with hopelessness is more dangerous, and suicidality increases markedly.[37] Depressive illness is potentially a fatal illness, particularly if associated with hopelessness and existential anxieties. Hopes are challenged by illnesses. Up to 45% of the dying struggle to maintain hope.[38] It is perhaps surprising in the presence of a poor prognosis, debilitating and fatal illness, fading hope and a depression prevalence of 5–15%, that completed suicide is rare in cancer patients.

Suicidal thoughts occur in as many as 45% of terminally ill patients, though these are usually fleeting and often associated with feelings of loss of control and anxiety about the future.[39] Such thoughts provide a fantasised escape, a finality, from the current predicament. The will to live fluctuates substantially over hours and days in the terminal phase of life.[40] The desire for an early death is reported in 1.4%, 8.5% and 23% of terminally ill patients.[40–42] Depression was diagnosed in 17.6%, 58% and 100% of these patients.[40–42] In cancer patients with major depression (12.8% of the cohort), 51.4% expressed suicidal ideation.[43] Poor functional status and the severity of depression are significant risk factors for suicidal ideation. Pain is not an influence.[44] Depression and hopelessness are the strongest predictors of desire for death.[45] The existential state of mind of the patient may reinforce the death-seeking ideation. The demoralisation syndrome may progress to a desire to die or suicide.[29,31] Treatment of depression can diminish desire for death. A study of depressed geriatric patients' preference for life-sustaining therapy found that 25% showed an increased desire for such therapy after treatment of their depression.[46] This was particularly apparent in several of the most severely depressed patients. The desire to hasten death, however, is not necessarily synonymous with a request to hasten death.

Requests by patients to hasten death are relatively rare in palliative care practice. They are possibly commoner in other areas of medicine such as neurology, geriatrics and psychiatry. In the USA, 12% of physicians received one or more explicit requests in the previous year, and in a terminal care setting 7% of patients had asked.[47,48] In view of the frequency of the desire and the numbers of patients attended, it does appear that a sustained wish to die before nature determines is rather uncommon, unless depressed. Requests by relatives, often spontaneously and indirectly, are probably more frequent. The associations between depression and suicide, and depression and euthanasia requests, are evident. One must ask why so few patients commit suicide, and anecdotally they do not seem to be the same cohort of patients as those who discuss euthanasia.[49] Suicide is different from asking to be killed. They are differing expressions of an individual's control over life and destiny.

Management

A correct diagnosis of major depression allows one of the most confident estimations of response to treatment known to medicine. From the clinical perspective a crucial decision is whether or not to introduce biological interventions.

With the emerging trend of the over-prescription of antidepressant medication, for these medications are tolerable and cheap (in comparison to psychotherapy), the temptation is to diagnose positively in the 'grey' or marginal cases. However medications have both physiological and psychological adverse effects and they do not work in mild and reactive depressive syndromes.

The initial clinical task is to ensure the patient is safe, in a secure environment with careful ongoing monitoring. Suicidal ideation is an intensely personal matter. Yet those harbouring such thoughts may be relieved that someone bothers to inquire about their intent, plan and access to means. Such questioning is unlikely to prompt the patient to consider suicide, however it is advisable to introduce the topic gently. For example 'have you thought you may be better off dead?'. In the terminally ill, attending to associated uncomfortable symptoms of their primary illness, such as pain, is critical. Adequate analgesia alone improves wellbeing if not mood. Nausea is a most distressing symptom and creates despair and desperation. For those previously physically active and energetic, the fatigue of cancer may seem intolerable. Establishing a therapeutic alliance, initiated by an empathic and sensitive assessment interview, encourages sufficient trust to commence discussion about the required treatment modalities and options. A psychological intervention is mandatory, whereas physical treatment interventions should be reserved for moderate and severe depression. Initially psychoeducation about depressive disorders is necessary, and indeed this process is really the introduction of psychotherapy.

Psychotherapy

Psychotherapeutic interventions need to be matched to the condition and to the individual. In mild depression and reactive dysthymia, merely acquiring the history may be sufficient. The clarification of stressors, the offering of empathy and understanding may allow the patient to forthwith regain coping and competency. Information about the condition and its expected prognosis may be reassuring. The anxiety of 'going crazy' and 'out of control' is a fundamental fear for everyone. Consultation–liaison psychiatrists spend much of their time diagnosing 'sanity' and 'sadness' in the physically ill.

Physical touch is soothing both for body and mind. Nursing staff can easily capitalise on this and very rapidly establish a (psycho)therapeutic relationship. Relaxation therapies and many complementary treatments involve distraction, physical loosening, and reinforcement of simple task competency. 'Psychologising' personal problems is very much a Western concept. Most people of the world portray distress in a physical modality, and it responds well to somatic interventions, albeit transiently. Psychotherapy has acquired a reputation as therapy provided only by specifically trained experts. For the physically frail, such talking therapies are often neither feasible nor effective. Potentially the most potent psychotherapist for the dying is the attending nurse, for she has jurisdiction over the patient's physicality. Her reassurances and esteem building can prove the foundation upon which the depression lifts.

Patients in the 'grey zone', in whom some minor and variable physiological symptoms of depression may be present, may require a more formalised psychotherapeutic approach. Short-term supportive psychotherapy (perhaps

4–10 sessions), based on a crisis intervention model, should be provided. The aim of therapy is to enhance morale and self-esteem while decreasing distress and improving coping methods or strategies.[50] Reinforcing self-worth by emphasising past strengths and previous successful ways of coping, correcting negative misconceptions and cognitions, addressing current interpersonal conflicts and supporting adjustment to the limitations imposed by the disorder are some of the core tasks of therapy. Poor social supports, social disconnection and isolation compound coping difficulties. Involving family is often advisable and certainly they need information and support. Cognitive–behavioural therapy (CBT), interpersonal therapy (IPT), analytic psychotherapy and a vast array of talking therapies all have clinical advocates. Cognitive therapies involving reframing and restructuring of negative thought patterns can help shift passive helplessness to a more active coping style. The necessary basic ingredients of all such therapies include empathy, interest and support over a time-limited period. Termination of therapy is a component of the treatment, and this is as important in the dying as it is for all. Cathartic psychotherapies are popular. They seem comprehensible to many, for 'getting things off one's chest' appeals, they don't demand any internal change or accommodation, therefore the distress soon recurs. Impending death can serve as a powerful psychological tonic. Rapid and meaningful resolution of personal and family dynamics can occur. There are studies suggesting that psychosocial interventions result in longer survival, perhaps because of improved adherence to medical care. However there is no literature on the effectiveness of psychotherapy on depressive, rather than distressing, symptoms.[5,51]

Melancholic patients also require good supportive psychotherapy. The focus needs to be pragmatic and educational about the disease 'depression', and compliance with medication. Procrastination needs to be advocated, for ill persons should delay in making major life-determining decisions, until well. Guidance and distinct advice for these patients may be required in the interim until they recover sufficiently to resume autonomous functioning. Medical paternalism can be both benign and therapeutic.

Pharmacotherapy

The major clinical decisions with respect to choosing an antidepressant are those of the symptom profile, adverse reactions and the required onset of action. There is little if any efficacy difference across the range of available antidepressant medications. Antidepressant medications treat MDD successfully in 65% of cases.[3] SSRI, TCA and MAOI antidepressants all have a 60–70% response rate in the otherwise physically well. However the response rate in organic depressions is closer to 40%.[52] Psychostimulant response rates are around 50%. Increasingly it is recognised that the type of affective symptom suggests the appropriate and effective medication. Parker's model of symptom profile determining antidepressant choice is useful.[8] A serotonergic medication should be used for anxious depression, a noradrenergic antidepressant for retarded or melancholic depression, and if psychosis is a feature then an antipsychotic medication should be added.[8] In those with previous effective antidepressant use it is sensible to recommence this particular medicine.

The choice of medication in the terminally ill is influenced by co-morbid conditions and adverse reaction profile. Antidepressant medication may have analgesic actions (*see* Chapter 4), interact with analgesia (e.g. SSRI and codeine), assist sleep, and anticholinergic side-effects may assist continence. They may aggravate an already dry mouth, cause nausea and diarrhoea, blurred vision, and induce bladder spasm, a serotonin syndrome or delirium. Physically ill patients are particularly prone to, and troubled by, medication adverse reactions. The adverse effects of medications are not only physiological. Introducing psychotropic medication, particularly if the diagnosis is uncertain, tends to psychologically undermine already strained coping strategies. The implicit message of prescribing is 'you can't recover with your own resources, you need chemical help'. Actually this is incorrect for most affective disorders. Antidepressant medications merely enhance the rate of recovery, for eventually, at indeterminate time (from 6 months to decades), depressions tend to spontaneously remit. Many patients perceive the introduction of antidepressants as a personal failure. Adding to the burden of dis-ease associated with their primary disorder, medication adverse reactions are likely to dissuade compliance. Drug–drug interactions may occur as therapies change. Tamoxifen-associated reduction of TCA levels in blood has been reported.

There are undoubted barriers to the prescribing of antidepressant medications in palliative care settings. These include under-recognition of depression, lack of clinical knowledge and prescriber confidence, the stigma of psychiatric illness, the focus on other symptoms, the fear of compounding the patient's distress, and a sense of therapeutic nihilism in the dying.[39] Only one-third of 150 clinically depressed cancer patients actually were prescribed antidepressant medications in a recent Scottish study,[53] and 32% (mostly an SSRI) in another.[42] A 30% increase in psychotropic prescribing over a 10-year period has been documented.[54] While these figures are an improvement on earlier studies they still suggest undertreatment. Educating oncologists to prescribe antidepressants (fluoxetine) utilising a brief assessment tool and a simple treatment algorithm was shown to result in uniform improvement in a group of their patients.[55] Educating non-psychiatrist colleagues is obviously the most likely successful strategy to improve the recognition and appropriate treatment of depression. Clinicians should have a low threshold for initiating treatment.[39] Because of the enhanced propensity of the medically ill to experience adverse reactions of psychotropic medications, and a tendency for response to occur at lower doses, antidepressants should be 'started low and go slow'.

The duration of expected life in the terminally ill is a very relevant influence upon antidepressant choice. The rate of therapeutic onset of antidepressant medications has long been of clinical concern and dubious industry claims. It is generally accepted that there is a lag between the necessary therapeutic dose and clinical response of 1–2 weeks, and for some patients 4–6 weeks irrespective of the particular compound. This may be incorrect, and response can occur within days for some.[56] Prior to improvement of mood in medication-responsive patients, a transient and potentially dangerous jag of enhanced anxiety may occur. This is probably a mild serotonin syndrome induced by the medication. It settles over 24–48 h, and its intensity is relieved by benzodiazepines. Florid serotonin syndromes may rarely occur with medications and combinations that enhance serotonin activity. Within hours the patient may develop agitation, a hyperaroused state, myoclonus, hyperreflexia, diaphoresis and disturbance of consciousness. Normality returns usually within 72 h, with cessation of the medication and supportive care. Conventional clinical opinion is that a thera-peutic trial generally takes 4–6 weeks. For the terminally ill this lag may preclude the use of conventional antidepressants, hence the role for psychostimulants.

The effectiveness of combined psychological–pharmacological therapy in physically well adults is impressive, in the vicinity of 70–80%. Effectiveness of antidepressants has been shown in depressed cancer patients,[5] though definitive evidence is limited.[47] There is insufficient evidence-based information in hospice and terminally ill patients to confirm such good response rates. However it would be surprising in view of the knowledge that organic depressions are less responsive to treatment and most terminally ill patients have relevant organic aetiological influences upon their mood. TCAs in a cohort of medically ill patients (some of whom had cancer) resulted in only a 40% response rate.[52] Once initiated, antidepressants in the terminally ill generally should be continued indefinitely. The exception to this may be psychostimulants. A short 2–3-week pulse of this treatment can be sufficient to lift a depression and initiate neuro-transmitter recovery. However dose may require adjustment with the emerg-ence of organ failure. Prophylactic antidepressant introduced prior to high-dose interferon-alpha therapy has been shown to prevent depression.[57]

Selective serotonin reuptake inhibitors (SSRIs)

Fluoxetine, available since the late 1980s, revolutionalised antidepressant pre-scribing. It is remarkably tolerable and safe. The gastrointestinal adverse reactions (nausea, anorexia, diarrhoea) occur in less than 10%, and insomnia, headache and drowsiness even less frequently. Nausea tends to emerge early and abate quickly, though if this does not happen after several days (and anti-emetics rarely help), cessation needs to be considered. Initial anxiety enhancement is to be anticipated and in the forewarned patient is rarely problematic. The concerns regarding an increase of suicidality have been over-emphasised. All effective antidepressants lift mood and enhance energy and purpose, and suicidal risk can be anticipated to also increase transiently. Comparing this minute risk to the rate of suicide in untreated depression (about 50% attempt suicide) needs to be incorporated into the risk–benefit decision-making of the clinician. The sero-tonergic syndrome is rare, unless combined with another serotonin-acting com-pound (including St John's Wort). The sexual adverse reactions are of concern, even in a terminally ill population, as is the risk of inappropriate antidiuretic hormone secretion. SSRIs are effective as TCAs. Fluoxetine is available in tablet and capsule forms. The contents of the capsules can be dissolved in water and aliquots of smaller doses can be measured out, if the liquid preparation is unavailable. This may be very helpful in those having difficulties swallowing. An advantage as well as a disadvantage of fluoxetine and its active metabolite is the long half-life of 7–9 days (though metabolites may last in the system for weeks). This allows infrequent dosing regimes (and better compliance), but if intolerable it creates lengthy adverse effects. Drug interactions are problematic with fluoxetine. All so-called 'antidepressants' are effective anxiolytic medica-tions, perhaps more effective than they are antidepressants. More recently developed SSRIs, particularly citalopram, escitalopram and sertraline, are pre-ferable for use in the physically ill as they are slightly better tolerated and virtually free of drug interactions.

Tricyclic antidepressants (TCAs)

The most commonly used TCAs are the tertiary amines (amitriptyline, doxepin) and the secondary amines (nortriptyline, desipramine). Seemingly because of its use in the management of neuropathic pain, amitriptyline is a frequent choice. It is viciously toxic in the medically frail. The adverse reactions include anticholinergic effects (dry mouth, constipation, tachycardia, postural hypotension, blurred vision, urinary retention and delirium), arrhythmias, orthostatic hypotension and sedation. It increases the risks of falls threefold. In medically ill patients (including some cancer patients), 32% had to withdraw from the medication because of adverse reactions (delirium 16%, urinary retention 4%).[52] Amitriptyline's active ingredient is nortriptyline, which is a very much better tolerated medicine. Nortriptyline should be commenced at 5–10 mg nocte and slowly titrated upwards until a reasonable sleep is achieved, without daytime sedation. This is usually about the therapeutic dose. In physically healthy adults the therapeutic dose is 75–125 mg nocte. Particularly in debilitated patients, low dosage regimes tend to be effective. Serum levels of nortriptyline, unlike the other tricyclics, are an accurate indicator of therapeutic and toxic ranges. Drug–drug interactions, particularly with antihypertensive regimes and sedatives, should be monitored. TCAs can be administered as rectal suppositories if the oral route is not possible. Parenteral forms have been used but are not easily available.

Psychostimulants

Psychostimulant medication has a distinct role in palliative care. Used in North America to counteract the sedation associated with high-dose opioid analgesia and augment opioid analgesic regimes,[58] they also have an important place in the management of depression associated with advanced physical illness. Anxiety can also be improved by psychostimulants, a phenomenon (with smoking) known as Nesbitt's paradox. Clinical responses to stimulant medications are devious. In normal subjects initial drowsiness occurred in 50–65%,[59] and this is also recognised with caffeine. A beneficial and alerting response to caffeine, which occurs in about one-third of users (as does sedation), can be a clinical clue that a response to a stimulant may eventuate.[60] Six cups of coffee (600 mg caffeine) is roughly equivalent to 5 mg amphetamine.[61] Alertness to stimulants only occurs in 33–50%. The effectiveness of stimulants is greatest when the subject is sleepy (or perhaps physically frail). The onset of action of psychostimulants is rapid, usually within 24–48 h. Obviously this is of tremendous advantage in the terminally ill. There appear to be no established differing clinical effects of dexamphetamine and methylphenidate. Pemoline has been withdrawn for safety reasons (cardiac malformation risks). There are no robust clinical trials to support the effectiveness of psychostimulants in depressive disorders, but anecdotally it seems as if it may be in the vicinity of about 50%, significantly less than with conventional antidepressants. However in the physically ill psychostimulants may be at least as effective as conventional antidepressants, if not more so. In cancer patients, 83% showed some improvement within 48 h of commencement, and only 10% discontinued due to adverse reactions.[62] Doses of methylphenidate up to 20–30 mg/day are usually adequate. For psychiatric indications such as attention deficit hyperactivity disorder (ADHD), methylphenidate 1 mg/kg may be used, however this appears not to be necessary when used as an anti-depressant. They are generally well tolerated. Headache, agitation and rest-lessness may occur and delirium is a documented risk (particularly in demented individuals), though such medications have been advocated for hypoactive deliria. Cardiac arrhythmia is a relative contraindication, as resting pulse rate is slightly increased, though psychostimulants are safer than tricyclics for the heart. Only with chronic use (at >50 mg amphetamine/day), very high dosage (100–300 mg amphetamine/day) and in schizophrenic patients is there a risk of paranoid psychosis. Doctors tend to overestimate the adverse effects of psycho-stimulants, probably because of limited prescribing experience. Because of their activating action, psychostimulants should be administered early in the morning. They may additionally improve energy and appetite.[63] In contrast to their use as an appetite suppressant in the young diet conscious female, in the physically ill they tend to motivate appetite. While diversion needs to be considered, the risks of dependence and addiction in the physically ill are negligible. The duration of use needs to be determined by trial and error. Many organic depressions respond with a pulse of 2–3 weeks of psychostimulant, some require an ongoing regime. Dose escalation/tolerance appears not to be a problem, except in those with substance abuse histories. In persons with expected longevity, commencing a conventional SSRI concurrently is safe, and when the antidepressant therapeutic activity kicks in, the stimulant can be ceased. There are suggestions that efficacy of psychostimulants may fade in the last days of life,[64] as the dopamine and noradrenaline levels are too depleted to be able to be released. Modafinil may assume the mantle as the preferred psychostimulant for it appears to have no reported abuse potential.

Other antidepressant medications

MAOIs tend not to be used because of interaction risks. Moclobemide, par-ticularly if effective in a prior depressive episode, may be used, for interactions are unlikely. Trazadone is a useful hypnotic but has unpredictable antidepressant efficacy. Venlafaxine is a serotonin–noradrenaline reuptake inhibitor (SNRI). At doses less than 225 mg/day it is a conventional SSRI, at higher doses it is dual acting. It may have a particular role in neuropathic pain. Mirtazapine is a nor-adrenaline and specific serotonin antagonist (NaSSA). It is fast acting, virtually devoid of anticholinergic adverse reactions, sedating, an appetite stimulant, and an anti-emetic. It is used increasingly as a co-analgesic in chronic pain, and may assume a role as an alternative to the TCAs in this setting.

Other treatments

Electroconvulsive therapy (ECT)

The safest and most effective of the antidepressant therapies, ECT, is rarely a possibility for the severely medically ill. The major risks of ECT are those of the general anaesthetic. However the treatment option should not be dismissed for it can be a magical intervention for severe suicidal and psychotic depressions.

Phototherapy

Three terminally ill patients, without seasonal affective disorder, were reported to respond within days to exposure to bright wide-spectrum light.[65]

Complementary therapies

These may promote wellbeing and perhaps be of benefit to depressed terminally ill patients.[66]

References

1   Ovid. Tristia. iv, vi. 43. *Ovid with an English Translation: Tristia, Ex Ponto.* AL Wheeler. London: William Heinemann; 1959, p. 189.

2   Brugha TS. Depression in the terminally ill. *Br J Hosp Med.* 1993; 50: 176–81.

3   American Psychiatric Association. Treatment will lesson suffering, yield significant cost savings. *Psychiatric News.* 1993; April 16: 4.

4   Croyle RT. Depression as a risk factor for cancer: renewing a debate on the psychobiology of disease. *J Natl Cancer Inst.* 1998; 90: 1856–7.

5   Evans DL, Charney DS, Lewis L *et al.* Mood disorders in the medically ill: scientific review and recommendations. *Biol Psychiatry.* 2005; 58: 175–89.

6   Cowper W. *Charity.* I.159. In: *The Oxford Book of Quotations: Third Edition.* London: Book Club Associates; 1981, p. 164.

7   Burton R. *The Anatomy of Melancholia.* Pt.I, Sec.3, Mem.I, Subs.4. New York: New York Review of Books; 2001, pp. 406–7.

8   Parker G. Classifying depression: should paradigms lost be regained? *Am J Psychiatry.* 2000; 157: 1195–203.

9   Musslmann DL, Miller AH, Porter MR *et al.* Higher than normal plasma interleukin-6 concentrations in cancer patients with depression: preliminary findings. *Am J Psychiatry.* 2001; 158: 1252–7.

10 Hardman A, Maguire P and Crowther D. The recognition of psychiatric morbidity on a medical oncology ward. *J Psychosom Res.* 1989; 33: 235–7.

11 Maguire P. Barriers to psychological care in the dying. *BMJ.* 1985; 291: 1711–13.

12 Cochinov H, Wilson K, Enns M *et al.* 'Are you depressed?' Screening for depression in the terminally ill. *Am J Psychiatry.* 1997; 151: 674–6.

13 Lloyd-Williams M, Dennis M, Taylor F *et al.* Is asking patients in palliative care, 'Are you depressed?' appropriate? Prospective study. *BMJ.* 2003; 327: 372–3.

14 Johnson S. Quoted by James Boswell in *The Life of Samuel Johnson.* Harmondsworth: Penguin; 1986, p. 231.

15 Wilhelm K, Mitchell P, Slade T *et al.* Prevalence and correlates of DSM-IV major depression in an Australian national survey. *J Affect Dis.* 2003; 75: 155–62.

16 Hotopf M, Chidgey J, Addington-Hall J *et al.* Depression in advanced disease: a systematic review Part I. Prevalence and case finding. *Palliat Med.* 2002; 16: 81–97.

17 Cochinov HM, Wilson KG, Enns M *et al.* Prevalence of depression in the terminally ill: effects of diagnostic criteria and symptom threshold judgments. *Am J Psychiatry.* 1994; 151; 751–7.

18 Massie MJ, Gagnon P and Holland JC. Depression and suicide in patients with cancer. *J Pain Symptom Manage.* 1994; 9: 325–40.

19 Conill C, Verger E, Henriquez I *et al.* Symptom prevalence in the last week of life. *J Pain Symptom Manage.* 1997; 14: 328–31.

20 Coyle N, Adelhardt J, Foley KM *et al.* Character of terminal illness in the advanced cancer patient: pain and other symptoms during the last four weeks of life. *J Pain Symptom Manage.* 1991; 6: 408–10.

21 Minagawa H, Uchitomi Y, Yamawaki S, et al. Psychiatric morbidity in terminal cancer patients: a prospective study. *Cancer.* 1996; 78: 1131–7.

22 Nesse RM and Williams GC. Is depression an adaptation? *Arch Gen Psychol.* 2000; 57: 14–20.

23 van't Spijker A, Trijsburg RW and Duivenvoorden HJ. Psychological sequelae of cancer diagnosis: a meta-analytical review of 58 studies after 1980. *Psychosom Med.* 1997; 59: 440–3.

24 Cochinov HM, Tataryn DJ, Wilson KG *et al.* Prognostic awareness and the terminally ill. *Psychosomatics.* 2000; 41: 500–4.

25 Alexander PJ, Dinseh N and Vidyasagar MS. Psychiatric morbidity among cancer patients and its relationship with awareness of illness and expectation about treatment outcome. *Acta Oncologica.* 1993; 32: 623–6.

26 Lewis A. Melancholia: a clinical survey of depressive states. *J Ment Sci.* 1934; 80: 277–378.

27 Appels A and Mulder P. Excess fatigue as a precurser of myocardial infarction. *Eur Heart J.* 1988; 9: 758–64.

28 Engel GL. A psychological setting of somatic disease: the 'giving up–given up complex'. *Proc R Soc Med.* 1967; 60: 553–5.

29 Kissane DW, Clarke DM and Street AF. Demoralisation syndrome – a relevant psychiatric diagnosis for palliative care. *J Palliat Care.* 2001; 17: 12–21.

30 Kierkegaard S. *The Sickness Unto Death.* xi 132. In: Hong HV and Hong EH (eds). *The Essential Kierkegaard.* Princeton, NJ: Princeton University Press; 2000, p. 354.

31 Kissane DW and Kelly BJ. Demoralisation, depression and desire for death: problems with the Dutch guidelines for euthanasia in the mentally ill. *Aust N Z J Psychiatry.* 2000; 34: 325–33.

32 Allebeck P, Boland C and Rungback G. Increased suicide rate in cancer patients: a cohort study based on the Swedish cancer register. *J Clin Epidemiol.* 1989; 42: 611–16.

33 Crocetti E, Armiani S, Acciai S, Barchielli A and Buiatti E. High suicide mortality soon after diagnosis among cancer patients in Central Italy. *Br J Cancer.* 1998; 77: 1194–6.

34 Ripamonti C, Filberti A, Totis A, De Conno F and Tamburini M. Suicide among patients with cancer cared for at home by palliative care teams. *Lancet.* 1999; 354: 1877–8.

35 Breitbart W. Suicide in cancer patients. *Oncology.* 1987; I: 49–53.

36 Snowdon J and Baume P. A study of suicides of older people in Sydney. *Int J Geriatr Psychiatry.* 2002; 17: 261–9.

37 Uncapper H, Gallagher-Thompson D, Osgood NJ and Bongar B. Hopelessness and suicidal ideation in older adults. *Gerontologist.* 1998; 38: 62–70.

38 Radbruch L, Nauk F, Ostgathe C *et al.* What are the problems in palliative care? Results from a representative survey. *Support Care Cancer.* 2003; 11: 442–51.

39 Block SD. Assessing and managing depression in the terminally ill patient. *Ann Int Med.* 2000; 132: 209–18.

40 Cochinov HM, Wilson KG, Enns M *et al.* Desire for death in the terminally ill. *Am J Psychiatry.* 1995; 152: 1185–91.

41 Tiernan E, Casey P, O'Boyle C *et al.* Relations between desire for early death, depressive symptoms and antidepressant prescibing in terminally ill patients with cancer. *J R Soc Med.* 2002; 95: 386–90.

42 Brown J, Henteleff P, Barakat S *et al.* Is it normal for terminally ill patients to desire death? *Am J Psychiatry.* 1986; 143: 208–11.

43 Akecki T, Okamura H, Yamawaki S *et al*. Why do some cancer patients with depression desire an early death and others do not? *Psychosomatics*. 2001; 42: 141–5.

44 O'Mahony S, Goulet J, Kornblith A *et al*. Desire for hastened death, cancer pain and depression: report of a longitudinal observational study. *J Pain Symptom Manage*. 2005; 29: 446–57.

45 Breitbart W, Rosenfeld B, Pessin H *et al*. Depression, hopelessness, and the desire for hastened death in terminally ill patients with cancer. *JAMA*. 2000; 284: 2907–11.

46 Ganzini L, Lee MA, Heinz RT *et al*. The effect of depression treatment on elderly patients' preferences for life-sustaining medical therapy. *Am J Psychiatry*. 1994; 151: 1631–6.

47 Back A, Wallace J, Starks H *et al*. Physician assisted suicide and euthanasia in Washington State. Patient requests and physician responses. *JAMA*. 1996; 275: 919–25.

48 Emanuel EJ, Fairclough DL and Emanuel LL. Attitudes and desires related to euthanasia and physician assisted suicide among terminally ill patients and their caregivers. *JAMA*. 2000; 284; 2460–8.

49 Finlay I. From the UK. *Palliat Med*. 2003; 17: 137.

50 Holland J. Managing depression in patients with cancer. *CA Cancer J Clin*. 1987; 37: 366–71.

51 Williams S and Dale J. The effectiveness of treatment for depression/depressive symptoms in adults with cancer: a systematic review. *Br J Cancer*. 2006; 94: 372–90.

52 Popkin M, Callies A, Mackenzie T. The outcome of antidepressant use in the medically ill. *Arch Gen Psychiatry*. 1985; 42: 1160–3.

53 Sharp M, Strong V, Allen K *et al*. Major depression in outpatients attending a regional cancer centre: screening and unmet treatment needs. *Br J Cancer*. 2004; 90: 314–20.

54 Steifel F, Kornblith A and Holland J. Changes in the prescribing patterns of psychotropic drugs during a ten-year period. *Cancer*. 1990; 65: 1048–53.

55 Passik SD, Kirsh KL, Donaghy K *et al*. Use of a depression screening tool and a fluoxetine-based algorithm to improve recognition and treatment of depression in cancer patients: a demonstration project. *J Pain Symptom Manage*. 2002; 24: 318–27.

56 Posternak MA and Zimmerman M. Is there a delay in the antidepressant effect? A meta-analysis. *J Clin Psychiatry*. 2005; 66: 148–58.

57 Musselman DH, Lawson JF, Gumnick AK *et al*. Paroxetine for the prevention of depression induced by high dose interferon-alpha. *N Engl J Med*. 2001; 344: 961–6.

58 Bruera R, Fainsinger R, MacEachern T *et al*. The use of methylphenidate in patients with incident pain receiving regular opioids. A preliminary report. *Pain*. 1992; 50: 75–7.

59 Tecce JJ, Cole JO. Amphetamine effects in man: paradoxical drowsiness and lowered electrical brain activity (CNV). *Science*. 1974; 185: 451–3.

60 Rickels K, Ginrich RL Jr, Mclaughlin W *et al*. Metylphenidate in mildly depressed outpatients. *Clin Pharmacol Ther*. 1972; 13: 595–601.

61 Lader M. Comparison of amphetamine sulphate and caffeine citrate in man. *Psychopharmacologia*. 1969; 14: 83–94.

62 Olin J and Masand P. Psychostimulants for depression in hospitalised cancer patients. *Psychosomatics*. 1996; 37: 57–62.

63 Silverstone T. The clinical pharmacology of appetite – its relevance to psychiatry. *Psychol Med*. 1986; 47: 251–3.

64 Macleod AD. Methylphenidate in terminal depression. *J Pain Symptom Manage.* 1998; 16: 193–8.

65 Cohen SR, Steiner W and Mount BM. Phototherapy in the treatment of depression in the terminally ill. *J Pain Symptom Manage.* 1994; 9: 534–6.

66 Mermelstein H and Lesko L. Depression in patients with cancer. *Psychooncology.* 1992; 1: 199–215.

Chapter 7

Delirium

> When body is ill, soul goes awry often: it raves and utters foolishness, and sometimes lethargy weighs it down to deep and endless sleep.
>
> Lucretius (c99–c55 BC)[1]

Delirium is a common, if not inevitable, syndrome occurring during the final 24–48 h of life. Prevalence figures in the dying of up to 88% are quoted.[2] Delirium is a harbinger of death. It is under-recognised, under-treated and frequently mistreated.[3] To suffer delirium is frightening and distressing to both patient and staff.[4] The symptoms of delirium may be ameliorated and palliated even though its occurrence may be indicative of irreversible organ failure.

Conceptualising delirium

The term 'consciousness' in the DSM and ICD 10 diagnostic criteria for delirium (*see* Box 7.1) raises conceptual complexities, for it has differing medical and philosophical meanings.[5] The terms awareness, alertness, attention, arousal and awakeness have been used to clarify the meaning of 'consciousness', though they all remain difficult to independently define.[6] Consciousness is an amalgam of these separate but interconnected cerebral functions.

Impairment of consciousness is the primary and universal clinical change occurring in acute brain disease. Delirium lies on the continuum between full consciousness and deep coma. Consciousness is that state of an organism that enables cognitive processes to occur.[7] Delirium is best considered as primarily a disorder of alertness. Alertness refers to a state of enhanced readiness to receive and process information, and to respond.[8] When alert, stimuli are processed efficiently and responses initiated rapidly. To use a radio analogy, alertness

---

Box 7.1   DSM IV criteria for the diagnosis of delirium[5]

- Disturbance of consciousness (reduced clarity of environmental awareness) with impaired ability to focus or shift attention
- Change in cognition (memory impairment, disorientation, language disturbances, perceptual disturbances)
- Disturbance evolves over a short period of time (hours/days) and fluctuates during the course of the day
- Evidence of a general medical condition judged to be aetiologically related to the disturbance

---

represents 'volume'. To be alert, the brainstem needs to be functional. The predominant neurotransmitter involved is acetylcholine. Alertness is the 'key' that activates awareness. Awareness is the content of consciousness, it is higher mental functioning, and is dependent upon an intact cerebral cortex.[9] In radio terminology it is being 'in tune'. Arousal, or physiological readiness, is a more general term than alertness. It refers to an activated peripheral physiological state as well as to forebrain cortical activation.[7] High physiological arousal may or may not be associated with high levels of alertness, whereas low arousal tends to be associated with poor alertness. There is an obvious association between sleep and delirium. One needs to be awake to be conscious, yet the vegetative patient is 'awake but not aware'. The electroencephalogram (EEG) findings in delirium of generalised slowing are dissimilar to sleep. Delirium is but one of the disorders of consciousness. Dreaming, hypnosis, minimal conscious states and vegetative states are caused by differing impairments of these functions. At the bedside the level of alertness, or consciousness, can be crudely evaluated (*see* Box 7.2).

To the clinician the central concept is that of 'attention'. Attention is 'a control process that enables the individual to select, from a number of alternatives, the tasks he will perform or the stimulus he will process, and the cognitive strategy he will adopt to carry out these operations'.[10] Attention is the sentry gate of consciousness.[11] Alertness and awakeness are prerequisites for attention to occur. The importance of attention is that it may be objectively measured at the bedside. Inattention, distractability (the failure to select) and perseveration (the inability to shift attention) are key, though secondary or indirect, indicators of delirium. The pathological process of delirium is impaired alertness, and the clinical barometer of alertness is attention.[6]

The fundamental function of the brain is inhibitory, not excitatory. Its function is to suppress and organise the vast array of internal and external sensory stimuli (predominantly visual). If this processing and filtering is disrupted then

---

Box 7.2   Bedside indicators of delirium

- Level of consciousness:
  - full (alert, aware, attentive)
  - hyperalert/vigilant
  - hypoalert/drowsy
  - stupor/unrousable
  - coma
- Impairment of attention, as clinically assessed by:
  - disorientation in time (inaccuracy of greater than 1–2 h)
  - inability to recall examiner's name after 2 minutes
  - dysgraphic errors ('please write your home address'): omitted, reduplicated letters, misalignment, spelling, syntactical and dyslexic errors, hesitancy to write
  - inability to count down from 20 to 1
  - multiples of 2 (2×2, 2×4, 2×8 ... $2 \times 128 = 256$ is the usual normal range)
  - inability to recall 3 paired objects after 2 and 5 minutes

uncensored and chaotic cognitive, perceptual, affective and motor functioning result. Hughlings Jackson conceptualised nervous system functioning in evolutionary terms.[12] Upon damage to the CNS, dissolution of function occurs and behaviour reverts to that of an earlier (and intact) stage of development.[13] A loss of structure in the nervous system results in a compensatory increase of function of lower order structures. There is a reduction from the voluntary to the automatic, and from the complex to the simple. Damage to the nervous system 'releases' the inhibition over the remaining healthy tissue, and so-called 'positive' symptoms are expressed. Hence the diversity of symptoms. Damage to evolutionarily early structures, such as the brainstem, leads to downstream symptoms (impairment of awareness) and progressive biological withdrawal, a shutting down of the system (delirium, coma).

The syndrome

But for him it was his last afternoon as himself, an afternoon of nurses and rumours; the provinces of his body revolted, the squares of his mind were empty, silence invaded the suburbs, the current of his feelings failed; he became his admirers.

WH Auden (1907–1973)[14]

The acute onset of psychiatric symptoms in a person with compromised physical health is a necessary prerequisite for a diagnosis of delirium. There may be subtle prodromal symptoms such as restlessness, anxiety, insomnia, nocturnal muddledness and dreaming. The night nurse may the first to note these changes, for by day normality returns. The symptoms of established delirium are protean. Dysfunction of the brainstem results in consequential disorder in higher-level structure and function. Though the primary impairment is that of alertness, awareness is devastated because of this. All and every psychiatric and psychological symptom may occur. Thoughts and ideas lodged in memory are released, perceptual clarity is lost, and emotions spill out. Anxiety and fear are prominent. Impaired attention leads to disorientation (particularly to time). Retrieving recent memories and registering new memories results in distortions of memory and confabulation in an attempt to make sense of the world and prevent catastrophic reactions.[5] Sophisticated language functions deteriorate. Writing, a skill acquired relatively late in childhood and a symbolic representation of symbols (of sounds or speech) is vulnerable to error. Incoherent mutterings are common. Disorganised thinking, difficulties grasping one's circumstances and, literally, 'confusion' occur. Nominal aphasias are common, but not specific to delirium. Frank persecutory delusions may arise. Reasoning is defective. Visual, and less commonly olfactory, tactile and auditory illusions and hallucinations are indicative of the difficulties with alerting. Visual hallucinations occur in 40–75%, particularly in drug withdrawal deliria. These are highly variable and range from simple flashes of light to more discrete images. They tend to increase in darkness or upon closure of the eyes.[7] The sleep–wake cycle may be disrupted, sometimes reversed. Interpreting the content of psychotic symptoms in delirium is difficult. As in dreaming, there tends to be a component of the 'day's residue'.

There is, at least in the early phases of delirium, a fluctuation of the presence and intensity of symptoms. The clarity of the so-called lucid periods of delirium has not been quantified. Sundowning refers to the propensity for the aggravation of delirious symptoms as darkness falls, related partially to the loss of visual reminders but also to bodily temperature change.[15] Variations (of alertness) may be created by the inherent gamma or '40 Hz' rhythm of the brain. These episodic bursts of energy link the various regions of the brain in order to foster functional integration and to format information.[16] Alertness has a diurnal pattern, peaking in the morning. In Jacksonian terms the damage inflicted by the delirious insult results in regressive behaviour and primitive attempts to repair or heal. If, however, the toxic insult persists then there is no prospect of regeneration. With progression toward coma, fluctuations of mental status become less frequent and briefer.

Clinical assessment

The history of a recent change in mental status may be volunteered by the patient. Relatives and carers may provide compelling information and often describe a nocturnal onset of these changes.

At the bedside the key task is to evaluate alertness (*see* Box 7.2). Attention serves as an indirect barometer of alertness and awakeness. Inattention can be measured. An inability to direct, focus and sustain attention is usually apparent in the process of acquiring a history. Many bedside tests of attention, such as 100-7s, are not only excruciatingly difficult to explain to delirious persons, but are genuinely difficult tasks for most. Tests of cognition need to be simple and to extrapolate steeply in difficulty. Multiples of two is such a test involving an assessment of attention, concentration, recall and arithmetic dexterity. Reversal of the spelling of one's name, or a five-lettered word, and counting down from 20 to 1 are alternatives, the latter being the simplest. Traditionally, disorientation has been considered a relevant clinical sign of delirium. However orientation to time of day is the only valid test of orientation: day, date, month and year are of little relevance for watches or cell phones supply this information, supermarkets are open every day of the week, and sport is played most days of the year. It is surprising how often patients muddle mornings and afternoons. Misidentification of other people (usually mistaking the unfamiliar for the familiar) is a consequence of poor attention to detail or compromised registration. Paramnesia, the distortion rather than the loss of memory, is more typical than a global impairment of recent memory.[17] Many struggle to recall the examiner's name, let alone three paired objects after 2 minutes. Dysgraphia, while not specific for delirium, is not only a reasonably sensitive diagnostic aid, it is an easy serial assessment of clinical progress.[18] Bedside testing of constructional abilities such as the clockface test, if impaired does not distinguish delirium and dementia. However if normal, it is reasonable to conclude that the patient is not delirious. Testing cognitive functioning is invariably distressing for the patient.[19] It is bewildering to expose the deficits and may precipitate anxious and catastrophic reactions. Tests of cognition are best if brief and benign, and really serve only to support the clinician's clinical impression. Alone they are not diagnostically specific of delirium. The lack of clarity in thinking, literally confusion, is difficult to quantify and is not exclusive to delirium. The 'content' of consciousness, the symptoms of the 'final common neural pathway', are broad and non-specific to delirium, occurring in other psychotic, affective and anxiety states. Illusions, visual hallucinations, delusions, fear and moodiness are 'downstream' symptoms, and while deserving of management don't need to be quantified. Psychomotor behaviour is a gauge of the depth of consciousness impairment. The route to coma is that of initial hyperactivity (particularly if the cause is drug related), then hypoactivity (particularly if hepatic or metabolic in aetiology) and coma. Myoclonus can be considered a subtle motor sign of delirium, as is carphology (purposeless overactivity, picking at the bedclothes, groping movements). Brief and aggressive episodes of catatonic excitement, while unusual and unfortu- nately unpredictable, are dangerous. The sickest lose the capacity to arouse with behavioural activity as delirium deepens.

Diagnosing delirium is essentially that of a bedside clinical judgement. Criteria for uniformity, predominantly for research purposes, may be useful additions to clinical practice as screening and confirmatory tools. There is a multiplicity of such scales, all with attractions and limitations. The MMSE (Mini Mental State Examination) quantifies the impairments but doesn't distinguish delirium from dementia. The most useful tool is the Confusion Assessment Method (CAM see Box 7.3),[20] though the Delirium Rating Scale and the Memorial Delirium Assessment Scale have advocates. However the utility of such aids to diagnosis in the daily practice of palliative medicine are limited. Many patients have insufficient energy or interest to comply.

Box 7.3   The Confusion Assessment Method (CAM)[20]

- *Feature 1: acute onset and fluctuating course.* This feature is usually obtained from a family member or nurse and is shown by a positive response to the following questions: Is there evidence of an acute change in mental state from the patient's baseline? Did the (abnormal) behaviour fluc- tuate during the day, that is, tend to come and go, or increase or decrease in severity?
- *Feature 2: inattention.* This feature is shown by a positive response to the following question: Did the patient have difficulty focusing attention, for example, being easily distractible, or having difficulty keeping track of what was being said?
- *Feature 3: disorganised thinking.* This feature is shown by a positive response to the following question: Was the patient's thinking dis- organised or coherent, such as rambling or irrelevant conversation, with unclear or illogical flow of ideas, or unpredictable switching from subject to subject?
- *Feature 4: altered level of consciousness.* This feature is shown by any answer other than 'alert' to the following question: Overall, how could you rate this patient's level of consciousness? (Alert [normal], vigilant [hyper- alert], lethargic [drowsy, easily aroused], stupor [difficulty to arouse], or coma [unrousable].)

The diagnosis of delirium by CAM requires the presence of features 1 and 2 and either 3 or 4.

The physical signs of delirium vary to some extent upon aetiology. The presence of tachycardia, hypotension, flushing, sweating, diarrhoea, tremulousness, myoclonus and asterixis may hint at causes. In the frail elderly a febrile response to infection does not always occur. Reduced tissue turgor and mucosal dryness suggest dehydration. Pupillary size and examination of the optic fundi (if clinically possible) are unreliable signs in the dying patient. Primitive reflexes, focal neurology and meningism are suggestive of cerebral involvement. Myoclonus is a common generalised sign of nervous system toxicity.

Differential diagnosis

Testy delirium or dull decrepitude.

WB Yeats (1865–1939)[21]

All and every mental status aberration is possible in delirium. In the physically ill, delirium should be excluded as a diagnosis prior to formulating an alternative psychiatric diagnosis. Disturbance to consciousness does not occur in dementia, depression or schizophrenia. The diurnal fluctuations of mood in depressive disorders are of a consistent pattern rather than the rapidly changing, incontinent mood of delirium. Hypoactive delirium is liable to be mistaken for depression. The history of dementia is of gradual onset, and the impairments of longer-term memory, abstract thinking and higher cortical functions (aphasia, apraxia) are different. Demented patients are alert. Delirium is 2–3 times more common in the demented, the symptoms of delirium overshadowing those of dementia if these disorders co-exist. Fluent aphasic patients present a diagnostic challenge. They are more likely to produce neologisms and paraphasias in speech, and do not have attentional difficulties. The hallucinations of delirium are most commonly visual rather than the typical auditory hallucinations of schizophrenia. The delusions of delirium, most often paranoid in nature, tend to be more fragmented, less organised and more fleeting than those of schizophrenia.

Aetiology

In the terminally ill delirium is generally multidetermined (*see* Box 7.4). Intensive investigation provides specific causes in only 50%.[22] The absolute strength and activity of the noxious agent(s) and the host's vulnerability to such insult are the critical influences.[7] The interrelationship of precipitating and predisposing factors determines the clinical state (*see* Table 7.1). If vulnerability at baseline is low, patients may be resistant to delirium despite exposure to significant precipitating stressors, but if vulnerability at baseline is high, delirium is likely to occur with exposure to only minor precipitating factors.[23] Environmental influences may moderate these risks by muting the impact of the toxin and/or by strengthening the host. Individual differences in susceptibility to reacting with delirium to any given cause have been demonstrated.[7] Conceptualising delirium in terms of a 'threshold' model, a well-established model for epilepsy, is useful in understanding the various risk factors. The 'deliriant threshold' for each individual is unique.[6] The risk factors are multiplicative rather than additive. Limited 'brain reserve', as in the dementing or immature infant brain, enhances risks, as does the severity of the physiological insult. The physiological insult that eventually

---

Box 7.4   Causes of delirium in advanced cancer

Direct CNS involvement
- Primary tumour
- Brain metastases
- Post-ictal/seizures
- CNS infection

Systemic
- Organ failure:
  - hepatic encephalopathy
  - renal failure/uraemia
  - respiratory failure (pulmonary embolus, lymphangitis carcinomatosis, pulmonary oedema)
  - cardiac failure
- Electrolyte imbalance:
  - hypercalcaemia
  - hyponatraemia (rapidly occurring)
- Treatment-induced:
  - anticholinergic medications
  - opioids
  - corticosteroids
  - chemotherapy
  - radiotherapy
  - antiviral medication
  - anti-emetic medications
- Haematological
  - anaemia
  - disseminated intravascular coagulopathy
- Infection
- Nutritional
  - vitamin deficiency (Wernicke's encephalopathy)
- Paraneoplastic syndromes (limbic encephalopathy)

---

tips the patient into delirium may be in itself minor. Previous delirium increases the risk more significantly than does age and pre-existing cognitive impairment, suggesting a kindling effect.[24] Delirium is a syndrome of universal susceptibility.

Specific organic diseases don't give rise to specific delirium symptomatology. Iatrogenic causes are potentially reversible. Medications with anticholinergic effects in excess of 0.83 ng/ml of atropine-equivalent, are implicated in 20–40% of all deliria.[25] Opioids such as codeine (0.11 ng/ml atropine-equivalents), prednisolone (0.55 ng/ml atropine-equivalents) and, of course, antidepressants (particularly tricyclics) may lower the deliriant threshold.[25] The relationship of delirium and opioids remains uncertain. Anecdotally there does appear to be a chronological association on occasions, however in a prospective study of post-operative patients, delirium was nine times commoner in those deemed to have under-treated pain than those complying with opioids.[26] Nicotine withdrawal is

Table 7.1 Risk factors in delirium

Predisposing factors	Precipitating factors
Older age, very young age	Severe acute illness
Presence and severity of dementia	Infection
Previous delirium	Hyponatraemia
Functional dependence	Hypercalcaemia
Immobility	Hypoglycaemia
Dehydration	Hypoxia
Alcoholism	Renal failure
Severity of physical illness	Hepatic failure
? Genetics	Medication (opioids, tricyclics)
	Pain
	Anaemia
	Cerebrovascular disease
	Cerebral trauma
	Alcohol withdrawal
	Raised intracranial pressure
	Post-ictal state

usually countered if the patient is taking opioids. The not insignificant mortality of delirium tremens (DT) should persuade the clinician to treat on suspicion. Emergency treatment of DT with alcohol needs to be occasionally considered. Even at a late stage reversal may be possible in up to 50%, particularly if opioids and dehydration are implicated.[2]

Prevalence

Delirium is age related, though the symptoms are not age specific. Prevalence and incidence rates in cancer units have been reported as 45% and 42% respectively.[2] The incidence increases toward the approach of death. On admission to a palliative care unit 28–42% were experiencing delirium, a rate which increased to 88% before death.[2] If the road to coma is steep, then delirium may be passed through very rapidly. For most of those dying from cancer, the path to coma and death visits delirium. The prevalence of subsyndromal delirium may be substantial. One-third to two-thirds of deliria may be non-detected.[27] Nursing staff have been reported to have better detection rates than doctors, no doubt a feature of the length of direct patient contact involved in nursing as compared to the relative brevity of medical assessment.[28]

Investigations

Each medical investigation is associated with discomfort and/or risks. The only definitive diagnostic investigation for delirium is the EEG, which is not likely to be contemplated in the dying. A simple blood screen for blood count, electrolytes, glucose and calcium may provide clinically useful information. If infection is a possibility, urinalysis is warranted. The enthusiasm for investigation should be influenced by the stage of illness and the prospect of establishing a potentially reversible cause. Minimising iatrogenic discomforts such as that created by investigations requires sound clinical decision making. The confinement and the noise associated with MRI scanning, for example, may exclude this as an investigation option for the acutely delirious patient. Delirious symptoms can be amplified by such stressors. Clinical judgement, rather than laboratory tests, should determine treatment decisions. There is in palliative medicine no justification to investigate for medical curiosity alone.

Management

> Christ, may I die at night with the semblance of my senses, like the full moon that fails.
>
> Robert Lowell (1917–1977)[29]

The cardinal rules of management were formulated by medical writers of antiquity and these remain applicable today.[7] Diagnosis and management occur concurrently. Delirium requires therapeutic intervention beyond the identification of the syndrome and amelioration of the underlying cause. Box 7.5 lists the tasks of management in sequential and concurrent order.

Prevention and prophylaxis

Education of staff to ensure prompt recognition of delirium and multicomponent intervention strategies are effective measures reducing the duration and diminishing the severity.[30,31] Whether these strategies are truly preventative or prevent symptom escalation of subsyndromal delirium is uncertain.

The role of cytokines in delirium or, more particularly, the possibility that somatostatin and insulin-like growth factor-I (IGF-I) may prevent their rise, has resulted in them being postulated as potential neuroprotective agents against delirium.[32] Physical exercise is known to increase IGF-I uptake by the brain, thus supporting the purported protective role of exercise in delirium and suggesting an adaptive purpose of the hyperactivity of delirium.[33]

Prophylactic antipsychotic medication in patients at high risk, at least anecdotally, appears beneficial. Prophylactic haloperidol, given pre-operatively and continued postoperatively, has been shown to shorten the duration of delirium, but not its incidence.[34] Atypical neuroleptics deserve study in this regard. The preventative use of cholinesterase inhibitors similarly has appeal.[35]

Box 7.5   Principles of management

1   Prevention and prophylaxis
2   Creation of a safe environment
3   Treatment of the cause(s)
4   Palliation of medical symptoms
5   Environmental strategies
6   Psychological interventions
7   Pharmacological interventions

Creation of a safe environment

Delirium is a medical emergency. The initial priority is to minimise the risk of injury and harm to the patient, relatives, other patients and staff.[36] The symptoms are most easily containable within the familiarity of the home. The force of delusional ideation associated with delirium can provoke extraordinary physical strength, even in the elderly. The delusions of delirium tend to be poorly organised, transient, and readily influenced by environmental stimuli,[7] and counter-projective dialogue, while important, does not have the value it does in the more systematised and sustained delusions of schizophrenia. Counter-projective dialogue refers to the assumption of a neutral attitude, by neither agreeing nor disagreeing with the patient's ideation, yet empathising with the distress these thoughts must be causing them. Two-thirds of delirious patients were reported to have tried to, or had run away from hallucinatory images.[37] Perceptual release of visual imagery may be terrifying and dangerous. Organic psychoses are notoriously unpredictable, and the dangers may easily be under-estimated.

Informed consent for urgent interventions is often not attainable, unless a convenient lucid period presents. Emergency and life-saving interventions are governed by common law doctrine. Treatment may be given without informed consent if the treatment is such that medical colleagues would generally consider it appropriate, and a reasonable person would want it.[36] If the risk of injury to self and others is recurrent and persistent, and/or medical investigations and procedures are necessary, then utilising compulsory committal law is advisable, at least until the acute symptoms settle. Transferring such patients to a psychiatric ward is not appropriate, and may be dangerous because of the primary medical condition.[36]

Physical restraint, which requires at least five able-bodied staff members, should only be used if unavoidable, and only for very brief periods. The physical restraint of a delirious patient tends to increase agitation and paranoia,[36] and has been shown to increase the risk of deep vein thromboses, pulmonary emboli and cardiac arrhythmias.[38] The use of bed rails should be avoided as they merely increase the height of the potential fall without reducing the risk of the fall. Placing the patient's mattress on the floor is a safe, but admittedly undignified, option to increase the level of physical safety. The removal of dangerous objects and possible weapons (such as cutlery) is a necessary precaution.

Diffusing and calming techniques should be practised. A wandering patient may be managed by collusion, that is walking with the patient and generally redirecting them. Confrontation, the invasion of the patient's personal space and 'eyeballing' are best avoided as they are provocative. The effects of calming practices are not easily quantified, but anecdote and opinion suggest they certainly reduce behavioural escalation and violence in delirious persons.

Treatment of the cause(s)

Overall reversibility rates of delirium are determined predominantly on whether or not the causes are amenable to medical intervention. After correction of the cause, resolution of the mental state may take several days. Toward the last few days of life, reversal is less likely, for disease burden is considerable. However some interventions even at a late stage may be very effective. Antibiotic treatment of a minor infection, opioid rotation, and adequate analgesia are such examples. Medication regimes with marked anticholinergic activity may be reversed by procholinergic agents such as physostigmine and cholinesterase inhibitors.

Palliation of medical symptoms

Antipyretic medications and cooling are of effect reducing fever, oxygen may be helpful in hypoxic patients, and analgesia may ease discomfort. Even when the aetiology cannot be reversed, interventions that partially ameliorate the causes should decrease the intensity of the delirium, e.g. managing anaemia with blood transfusions or erythropoietin, raised intracranial pressure with corticosteroids and hypercalcaemia with bisphosphonates. In the short term, fluid intake is more important than nutrition (though solid food is a more efficient provider of hydration). A subcutaneous infusion of 1–2 l of fluid overnight may be an option to hydrate, although lines may be extracted by the muddled patient. Nasogastric feeding is not recommended as it is unpleasant and patients frequently wrench such tubes out. Urinary retention may require urinary catheterisation, and attending to constipation is an important consideration.

Environmental strategies

Therapeutic manipulations of the environment are under-utilised interventions and free from adverse effects.[39] Noisy, unfamiliar and unwelcome perceptual stimuli further compound the existing impairment of sensory filtering in the reticular activating system (RAS) of delirious patients, thus amplifying delirious symptoms. A failing brain, like an ailing heart, benefits from the reduction of its workload, hence the desirability to restrict, but possibly not deprive, the sensory input. A moderate sensory balance and an unambiguous environment are preferable to sensory over-stimulation.[36,39] Defective perceptual discrimination facilitates the occurrence of distortions and misinterpretations of sensory stimuli in busy environments.[7] Light is the preferable environment for delirium, and certainly in those in whom visual misperceptions are common the room should be well lit.[19]

The noise level should be below 45 dB during the day and less than 20 dB at night.[33] Limiting staff interactions with the patient, minimising staff changes and restricting visitors are important. Constancy of staff may be difficult to achieve, and the theoretical advantages of nursing patients in quiet side rooms must be weighed against the risk of nursing neglect.[39] The presence of personal artefacts and objects may reduce the unfamiliarity of a hospice environment. A later acrophase of high core body temperature is implicated in the sundowner effect in Alzheimer's patients.[15] The room temperature should be kept between 21.1 degrees Celsius and 23.8 degrees Celsius.[33] A bland and simple environment reduces the perceptual load on the brain.

Psychological interventions

Psychological interventions are under-utilised, yet are easy and anecdotally effective.[40] Nursing staff and supportive relatives are best placed to use such strategies as simple and firm communication, taking advantage of any lucid moments, and repetition of any information provided. Continual reassurance, orientation, explanation and clarification result in some relief of fear and bewilderment, albeit transiently. Holding the patient's hand is an effective means of focusing their attention and providing reassurance.[39] The inherent fear of the loss of sanity is difficult to check, for delirium is indeed insanity. That this state is nearly always temporary and interspersed with episodes of sanity should be emphasised. The use of the patient's name can be an important point of reference for the confused patient. Speaking slowly and using careful and distinct diction may help.[39] Fostering the individual's sense of control and competency, where possible, is important.[33] The simple opportunity to clean one's own teeth helps retain and regain a semblance of dignity and autonomy. The attendance and the assistance of close relatives, while ideal, can be counter-therapeutic if the relative is anxious or frightened.[33] Delirium, by its very nature, virtually precludes the conducting of counselling and psychotherapy, and it hinders the patient's ability to participate and to be involved in therapeutic decision-making. It destroys any meaningful communication for much of the time. Abreactive and explorative techniques are contraindicated.

Pharmacological interventions

Non-pharmacological treatments should not be abandoned with the introduction of medication, indeed they should be practised with renewed vigour, for the patient is likely to be increasingly responsive. The decision to administer drugs should not be influenced by the relative's wishes, time constraints or communication difficulties between medical and nursing staff, but by the patient's condition.[33] The benefits and the risks of adding medication to an already medically sick patient need to be considered carefully. Medications are more likely to be prescribed for frenetic, hyperactive delirium patients, because the disruption caused to others around them tends to demand intervention,[40] and non-pharmacological interventions may be impossible to practise because of the patient's gross inability to attend.

The intent of pharmacological intervention should be to alleviate the delirious symptoms (by tranquillisation), and if this is unsuccessful, to achieve a reasonable clinical outcome of minimising problem behaviour (by sedation).[33] Antipsychotic medications (also termed neuroleptic or major tranquilliser) calm, pacify, tranquillise or sooth by enhancing inhibition of sensory input. The 'workload' of the RAS is thus reduced, and the ensuing clinical consequence is the containment of the symptoms of delirium including agitated behaviour, psychosis and cognitive dysfunction, sometimes with the total amelioration of symptoms.[33] Antipsychotic medications are effective in both hyperactive and hypoactive deliria.[41] They generally improve cognition in both subtypes of delirious patients.[42] Sedative (or hypnotic) medications immobilise and induce (deep) sleep by depressing the level of consciousness. They carry a risk of worsening delirious symptoms at subhypnotic doses. Tranquillisation may need to be complemented with sedation, or on rare occasions a person may need to be chemically restrained by anaesthesia. Pharmacological antidotes may have a role if the aetiology is that of excess anticholinergic activity.

Antipsychotic medication

The medication of first choice for delirium is an antipsychotic. The mechanism of action of these medications in delirium is uncertain.[43] Maximal dopaminergic blockade occurs at relatively low doses and the rapidity of therapeutic onset of these agents (within hours) would suggest that this is not the mechanism of their action in delirium. Rebalancing the dopamine:acetylcholine ratio is a more compelling mechanism of action. A solitary randomised medication trial supports their use.[44]

There are particular forms of delirium in which antipsychotic medication is not the treatment of first choice. The use of benzodiazepines and/or a brief anticonvulsant regime is the treatment of choice for delirium tremens. Hepatic encephalopathy may be aggravated by the introduction of medications metabolised by the liver. AIDS and Lewy body dementia patients tend to be exquisitely sensitive to the neurological adverse effects of antipsychotic medications, thus benzodiazepines and cholinesterase inhibitors are the management options of choice. Animal studies indicate that antipsychotic medications may slow recovery after traumatic brain injury which is commonly complicated by delirium. The possibility of dangerous elongation of the QTc interval and the induction of torsades de pointes with antipsychotic medications needs to be considered in the benefit–risk equation.

Chlorpromazine and haloperidol have similar efficacy, however haloperidol is favoured for its preferable adverse effect profile and versatility of administration.[44] Haloperidol has few or no anticholinergic adverse effects, minimal cardiovascular effects, and its neurological adverse effects can be minimised by choosing the parenteral route of administration, such as the subcutaneous route.[45,46] Originally marketed as a 'stimulant antipsychotic', haloperidol is not sedating.[43] The efficacy, tolerability and safety have been demonstrated even at very high dose (*see* Box 7.6).[45] The neurological adverse effects of haloperidol peak at mid-range oral doses (5–20 mg). Administration of low dosage or high dosage (preferably parenterally) over a period of less than one month avoids the build up of the neurotoxic metabolite 'reduced haloperidol'.[45] In usual clinical practice the required dosage is only a few milligrams though doses of up to several hundred milligrams (intravenously) have been used with effect and safety. Haloperidol has suffered a mistaken reputation as a sedative and neurotoxic drug, however in experienced hands it remains the antipsychotic of first choice. Droperidol is no longer considered safe because of its propensity to prolongate the QTc interval more than many other antipsychotics. Chlorpromazine is painful when injected, and the risk of hypotension is significant. Levomepromazine, a potent phenothiazine, is used particularly if its major adverse effect, sedation, is desired to settle the agitated and restless patient. Risperidone may be the most frequently used atypical neuroleptic in delirium.[47] There are also clinical trial reports on the use of olanzapine and quetiapine.[48,49] Effectiveness in delirium is comparable to haloperidol (70–80% response rate), however sedation was a notable adverse effect and there are reports, particularly with olanzapine, of these medications aggravating or precipitating delirium.[50] Usefulness of these medications in the acute setting has been limited by the unavailability of short-acting parenteral options. Quetiapine may emerge as the most useful of these compounds for delirium.

Box 7.6 Intravenous haloperidol regime for acute delirium (adapted from Massachusetts General Hospital Guidelines)

- Initial dosage
  - mild symptoms: 1 mg
  - moderate symptoms: 5 mg
  - very severe symptoms: 10 mg
- Repeat and double dosage in 20–40 minutes if no control
- Repeat and double dosage each 20–40 minutes until clinical control achieved
- Await reappearance of symptoms and repeat last dosage
- Introduce oral dosing
- Phase out progressively as delirium clears

Note:
- 80% require <2 mg/24 h
- most settle within 1 h
- maximum single dose: 20 mg
- maximum daily dose: 100 mg

Sedative medication

Opium has been used since antiquity for its sedating effects, though tolerance to this adverse effect develops rapidly. Benzodiazepines are now the sedative drug of choice.[5] The induction of sleep in delirium may be crucial for the exhausted hyperactive patient in order to secure rest and safety. Benzodiazepines may reduce agitation in delirium, but they may also worsen cognitive impairment for they further lower consciousness and thereby aggravate delirium. To sedate, the required dose must be rapidly reached. Because of its very short half-life and speed of onset, midazolam is the benzodiazepine of choice. It is unlikely that there are distinct sedative efficacy differences between the benzodiazepines, and pharmacokinetic parameters should determine the choice. Their most clinically useful role is to safely augment antipsychotic medication and induce sleep and rest if required. The risk of a paradoxical behavioural response is small and predominantly related to pre-illness characteristics.[51] The failure to induce disinhibited behaviour even in a high-risk population suggests this concern is overstated.[52] Respiratory depression and arrest may occur with intravenous administration of benzodiazepines and needs to be considered as a risk. The safety of benzodiazepines in the medically ill is remarkable, and the availability of an antidote, flumazenil, is reassuring to the clinician, but rarely if ever necessary.

Anaesthesia

Deep sedation with respiratory support may rarely be required to control severe hyperactive deliria. Propofol at low dosage (10–50 μg/kg/min) has been used to anaesthetise these patients to enable treatment of the life threatening cause (such as acute viral encephalitis). Dexmedetomidine, a selective alpha$_2$-adrenergic receptor agonist, a novel anaesthetic agent, has also been trialled in postoperative delirium.[53]

Antidote medication

Dopamine–acetylcholine imbalance is postulated to be the central lesion in delirium. Acetylcholine decreases with age and is reduced in dementia. Many medications have significant anticholinergic activity.[27] Physostigmine (0.5–2.0 mg IV) rapidly reverses symptoms of anticholinergic delirium. The use of cholinesterase inhibitors in delirium in Lewy body dementia might also be considered an antidote intervention.[54]

Other pharmacological interventions

Psychostimulants such as methylphenidate have been used in hypoactive delirium to arouse and stimulate consciousness.[55] The 5HT$_2$ antagonist antidepressants mianserin and trazodone have been shown in open studies to rapidly reduce non-cognitive symptoms of delirium at low dose, this being independent of the mood-altering actions.[56]

Outcome

Rapid and full recovery is the desired outcome. A delay of up to several weeks in the 'high risk' persons, but a few days for most, is to be expected between abolishing the cause and the recovery of senses. In frail cancer patients, 68% were reported to have improved despite a 30-day mortality of 31%,[22] and rates of reversal of nearly 50% have been reported in such patients.[2] The outcome will depend upon the nature of the offending physiological stressor, the biological vulnerabilities of the patient and moderating environmental factors. The belief that full recovery generally occurred after delirium has been shown to be unlikely to be correct, especially in an elderly population. Enduring cognitive deficits, a subsequently lowered 'deliriant threshold' (hence the probability of future episodes), psychiatric morbidity and death may result. Complete symptom resolution was seen in only 52% of elderly hospitalised patients 12 months after delirium, and prolonged memory impairment was common in these patients.[57] Recollection of delirious episodes tends to be patchy (as would be expected with fluctuating cognitive and memory symptoms). These memories are distressing in 50%,[4] and the delirium experience has been reported to induce PTSD. The prevalence of accidental injury and suicide in delirium are not known. Mortality rates in the delirious hospitalised elderly range from 22% to 76%, and over 80% of those with terminal malignancy die delirious.[2] Historically delirium has been considered the harbinger of death.[7] In the palliative care patient population it should not be assumed that full recovery will occur even if the causes are reversible.

It is uncertain how effective interventions for delirium are. Clinically there is little doubt that significant palliation of symptoms is possible. In those cases in terminal care where the causes can't be reversed, and the symptoms are unable to be contained with multicomponent interventions (including pharmacological tranquillisation), deep sedation may be indicated (*see* Chapter 8). Dying is difficult, dying crazy is more difficult. Such 'bad' deaths may be preventable.

References

1 Lucretius. *The Nature of Things.* Book III, 463–6 (tr. FO Copley). New York: WW Norton; 1977, p. 77.

2 Lawler PG, Gagnon B Mancini IL *et al.* Occurrence, causes, and outcome in patients with advanced cancer. *Arch Intern Med.* 2000; 160: 786–94.

3 Inouye SK. The dilemma of delirium: clinical and research controversies regarding making diagnosis and evaluation of delirium in hospitalised elderly medical patients. *Am J Med.* 1994; 97; 278–88.

4 Breitbart W, Gibson C and Tremblay A. The delirium experience: delirium recall and delirium-related distress in hospitalised patients with cancer, their spouses/caregivers, and their nurses. *Psychosomatics.* 2002; 43: 183–94.

5 American Psychiatric Association. *Diagnostic and Statistical Manual of Mental Disorders* (4e). Washington DC: American Psychiatric Association; 1994.

6 Macleod AD. Delirium: the clinical concept. *Palliative and Supportive Care.* 2006; 4: 305–12.

7 Lipowski ZJ. *Delirium: acute brain failure in man.* Springfield: Charles C Thomas; 1980.

8 Brown VJ, Bowman ER. Alertness. In: Ramachandran VS (ed). *Encyclopedia of the Human Brain.* San Diego, CA: Academic Press; 2002, pp. 99–110.

9 Bateman DE. Neurological assessment of coma. *J Neurol Neurosurg Psychiatry.* 2001; 71(suppl 1): i13–i17.

10 Moscovitch M. Information processing and the cerebral hemispheres. In: Gazzaniga MS (ed). *Handbook of Behavioral Neurobiology, Neuropsychology.* Vol 2. New York: Plenum Publishing; 1979, pp. 379–446.

11 Zeman A. Consciousness. *Brain.* 2001; 124: 1263–89.

12 Dewhurst K. *Hughlings Jackson on Psychiatry.* Oxford: Sandford; 1982.

13 Power TD. Some aspects of brain–mind relationship. *Br J Psychiatry.* 1965; 111: 1215–23.

14 Auden WH. From 'In Memory of WB Yeats'. *Collected Shorter Poems 1927–1957.* London: Faber and Faber; 1966, p. 141.

15 Volicer L, Harper DG, Manning BC *et al.* Sundowning and circadian rhythms in Alzheimer's Disease. *Am J Psychiatry.* 2001; 158: 704–11.

16 Young BG and Pigott SE. Neurobiological basis of consciousness. *Arch Neurol.* 1999; 56: 153–7.

17 Geschwind N. Disorders of attention: a frontier in neuropsychology. *Phil Trans R Soc Lond B.* 1982; 298: 173–85.

18 Macleod AD and Whitehead LE. Dysgraphia and terminal delirium. *Palliat Med.* 1997; 11: 127–32.

19 Stedeford A. Understanding confusional states. *Br J Hosp Med.* 1978; 20: 694–704.

20 Inouye S, van Dyck C, Alessi C *et al.* Clarifying delirium: the Confusion Assessment Method. A new method for detection of delirium. *Arch Intern Med.* 1995; 155: 301–7.

21 Yeats WB. From 'The Tower'. *Collected Poems.* London: Picador; 1990, p. 224.

22 Bruera E, Miller L, McCallion J *et al.* Cognitive failure in patients with terminal cancer: a prospective study. *J Pain Symptom Manage.* 1992; 7: 192–200.

23 Inouye SK and Charpentier PA. Precipitating factors for delirium in hospitalised elderly persons. *JAMA.* 1996; 275: 852–7.

24 Litaker D, Locala J, Franco K *et al.* Preoperative risk factors for postoperative delirium. *Gen Hosp Psychiatry.* 2001; 23: 84–9.

25 Tune L, Carr S, Hoag E *et al.* Anticholinergic effects of drugs commonly prescribed for the elderly: potential means for assessing risks of delirium. *Am J Psychiatry.* 1992; 149: 1393–4.

26 Morrison RS, Magaziner J, Gilbert M *et al.* Relationship between pain and opioid analgesia on the development of delirium following hip fracture. *J Gerontol A Biol Sci Med Sci.* 2003; 58: 76–81.

27 Inouye SK, Bogardus ST Jr, Charpentier PA *et al.* A multicomponent intervention to prevent delirium in hospitalised older patients. *N Engl J Med.* 1999; 340: 669–76.

28 Gustafson Y, Brannstrom B, Norberg A *et al.* Underdiagnosis and poor documentation of acute confusional states in the elderly hip fracture patient. *J Am Geriatr Soc.* 1991; 39: 760–5.

29 Mariani P. *Lost Puritan: a life of Robert Lowell.* New York: WW Norton; 1994, p. 460.

30 Tabet N, Hudson S, Sweeney V *et al.* An educational intervention can prevent delirium on acute medical wards. *Age Aging.* 2005; 34: 152–6.

31 Milisen K, Lemiengre J, Braes T *et al.* Multi-component intervention strategies for managing delirium in hospitalised older patients: systemic review. *J Adv Nurs.* 2005; 52: 79–90.

32 Broadhurst C and Wilson K. Immunology of delirium: new opportunities for treatment and research. *Br J Psychiatry.* 2001; 179: 288–9.

33 Meagher DJ. Delirium: optimising management. *BMJ.* 2001; 322: 144–9.

34 Kalisvaart K. Prophylactic haloperidol cuts delirium. Paper presented at the Annual Meeting, American Geriatric Psychiatry, Honolulu, HI; 2003.

35 Dautzenberg PL, Wouters CJ *et al.* Rivastigmine in prevention of delirium in a 65 years old man with Parkinson's disease. *Int J Geriatr Psychiatry.* 2003; 18: 555–6.

36 Johnson MH. Assessing confused patients. *J Neurol Neurosurg Psychiatry.* 2001; 71(suppl 1): i7–i12.

37 Frieske DA and Wilson WP. Formal qualities of hallucinations: a comparative study of the visual hallucinations in patients with schizophrenia, organic and affective psychoses. In: Hock PH and Zubin J (eds). *Psychopathology of Schizophrenia.* New York: Grune and Stratton; 1966, pp. 49–62.

38 Gillick MR, Serrell NA and Gillick LS. Adverse consequences of hospitalisation in the elderly. *Soc Sci Med.* 1982; 16: 1033.

39 Lindesay J, Macdonald A and Starke I. *Delirium in the Elderly.* Oxford: Oxford University Press; 1990.

40 Meagher DJ, O'Hanlon D, O'Mahony E *et al.* The use of environmental strategies and psychotropic medication in the management of delirium. *Br J Psychiatry.* 1996; 168: 512–15.

41 Platt MM, Brietbart W, Smith M *et al.* Efficacy of neuroleptics for hypoactive delirium. *J Neuropsychiatry Clin Neurosci.* 1994; 6: 66–7.

42 American Psychiatric Association. Practice guidelines for the treatment of patients with delirium. *Am J Psychiatry.* 1999; 156(suppl): 1–20.

43 Vella-Brincat JB and Macleod AD. Haloperidol in palliative care. *Palliat Med.* 2004; 18: 195–201.

44 Brietbart W, Marotta R, Platt MM *et al.* A double blind trial of haloperidol, chlorpromazine and lorazepam in the treatment of delirium in hospitalized AIDS patients. *Am J Psychiatry.* 1996; 153: 231–7.

45 Sos J and Cassem NH. Managing post-operative agitation. *Drug Ther.* 1980; 10: 103–6.

46 Menza MA, Murray GB, Holmes VF *et al.* Decreased extrapyramidal symptoms with intravenous haloperidol. *J Clin Psychiatry.* 1987; 48: 278–80.

47 Schwartz TL and Masand PS. The role of atypical antipsychotics in the treatment of delirium. *Psychosomatics.* 2002; 43: 171–4.

48 Breitbart W and Tremblay A, Gibson C. An open trial of olanzapine for the treatment of delirium in hospitalised cancer patients. *Psychosomatics.* 2002; 43: 175–82.

49 Schwartz TL and Masand PS. Treatment of delirium with quetiapine. *Prim Care Companion J Clin Psychiatry.* 2000; 2: 10–12.

50 Lim CJ, Trevino C, Tampi RR. Can olanzapine cause delirium in the elderly? *Ann Pharmacother.* 2006; 40: 135–8.

51 Patton C. Benzodiazepines and disinhibition: a review. *Psychiatr Bull.* 2002; 26: 460–2.

52 Rothchild AJ, Shindul-Rothchild JA, Viguera A *et al.* Comparison of the frequency of disinhibition on alprazolam, clonazepam, or no benzodiazepine in hospitalised psychiatric patients. *J Psychopharmacol.* 2000; 55: 271–8.

53 Maldonado JR, van der Starre P, Wysong A *et al.* Dexmedetomidine: can it reduce the incidence of ICU delirium in postcardiotomy patients? (abstract). *Psychosomatics.* 2004; 45: 173.

54 Kaufer DI, Catt KE, Lopez OL *et al.* Dementia with Lewy bodies: response of delirium-like features to donepezil. *Neurology.* 1998; 51: 1512.

55 Stiefel F and Holland J. Delirium in cancer patients. *Int Psychogeriatr.* 1991; 3: 333–6.

56 Okamato Y, Matsuoka Y, Sasaki T *et al.* Trazodone in the treatment of delirium. *J Clin Psychopharmacol.* 1999; 19: 280–2.

57 Rockwood K. The occurrence and duration of symptoms in elderly patients with delirium. *J Gerontol.* 1993; 48: 162–6.

Chapter 8

Sleep, sedation and coma

When youth is wakeful and old age drowsy, death is nigh.

Ambroise Paré (1517–1590)[1]

Disturbances of sleep

Sleep is a state of 'suspended consciousness', a temporary interruption of sensorimotor interaction with the environment. Clinically the distinguishing feature of sleep, in contrast to coma, is the ease with which the sleeping subject can be roused to awareness of the external world. Normal sleep consists of two distinct phases. Normal sleep architecture is a continuous cycle, lasting approximately 90 minutes, of non-rapid eye movement (NREM) sleep and rapid eye movement (REM) sleep. The functions of sleep include rest and restoration, both physically and mentally. Stages 3 and 4 of NREM sleep (slow wave sleep, SWS) reorganise, update and repair the brain's synthetic processing or programming. An increase of immune activity also occurs during sleep.[2]

Total sleep time and time spent in SWS gradually decrease with age, and fragmentation of the pattern becomes more pronounced. Sleep efficiency is not proportional to the duration of sleep, and many elderly spend increased time in bed for lesser reward. The very elderly, and the profoundly ill, rest and sleep for longer periods, though the sleep doesn't refresh. Frequent daytime micronaps and a shorter night sleep are typical features. Clinically determining a patient's actual sleep is difficult. Lack of sleep tends to be over-estimated by most (pseudo-insomnia). A sleep diary and an interview with the bed partner and/or carer are the necessary sleep assessment tools. Polysomnography is seldom indicated, nor is it feasible. Affective disorder and chronic pain adversely affect sleep. Poor sleep is a contributing factor lowering the pain threshold, thus in palliative medicine sleep disorders merit serious attention.[2] Acute pain interrupts stage 2, NREM sleep, though how more chronic pain disrupts is less certain.[3] Sleep efficiency is reduced in chronic pain because of delayed sleep onset, frequent awakenings and alpha-delta intrusions into NREM.[4]

Insomnia

Insomnia is a common complaint of the terminally ill. In the general population difficulty getting off to sleep is reported by 10% of males and 18% of females aged 65 years or older, interrupted sleep in 23% and 28% respectively, and early morning wakening in 14%.[4] The prevalence in chronic pain and cancer patients is 50–70%.[5,6] Sleep deprivation has considerable effect on functioning. Mood, cognition and motor performances are adversely affected, and coping strategies

95

Table 8.1 Medications and sleep

	REM	SWS	NREM stage 2	Total sleep time	Sleep latency	Dreaming	Nightmares/ parasomnia	Fragmented sleep	Insomnia	Hypnotic effect
Opioids	↓	↓	↓	↑	↓	+		+		+
Benzodiazepine	↓	↓		↑	↓	+				+
Non-benzodiazepine hypnotic	↓	↑	↑		↓					+
Tricyclics	↓	↓	↑	↑	↓	±	+			+
SSRIs	↓			↓		±	+		+	
Antipsychotics	↓			↑	↓		+			+
Anticonvulsants	↓	↑	↑	↑	↓			+		+
L-dopa	↓	↓				+	+	+	+	
Psychostimulant	↓	↓		↓	↑			+	+	
Alcohol	↓	↑		↓	↑			+	+	
Corticosteroid	↓	↓	↑		↑	+	+		+	
NSAIDs	↓			↓	↑			+	+	
Beta-blockers	↓					+	+		+	

±: dreaming occurs at subtherapeutic doses.

are seriously undermined. The onset and maintenance of sleep are not passive processes. A combination of cerebral competency and good habits are required. Sleep disturbance in critically ill patients is due to the noisy and intrusive environment, the medications used (*see* Table 8.1) and the disease (particularly if respiratory).[7]

The pattern of the insomnia indicates possible aetiology. Initial insomnia, the inability to fall asleep when desired in the evening, is the most common form of insomnia. Sleep hygiene habits such as a regular bedtime, avoidance of caffeine and fluids over early evening, using bed for sleep and intimacy only (and not TV or reading), mild exercise, and a warm milk drink on retiring may all be upset by the inconveniences of illness. Opportunities to sleep during the day induced by fatigue and boredom also unsettle habitual rhythms. An unfamiliar (hospice) bed, differing temperature, noise and lighting levels all may contribute negatively (or beneficially). Unrelieved symptoms of illness such as pain, dyspnoea, vomiting, itch and diarrhoea are liable to interfere with sleep initiation. Corticosteroid, diuretic, psychostimulant and sympathomimetic medications, and alcohol or benzodiazepine withdrawal states, can disrupt the onset of sleep. Very short-acting hypnotics can result in rebound prior to morning. Akathisia, induced by anti-emetics or antipsychotics, can escalate nocturnally. Hiccups tend to disappear at sleep onset (though they can disrupt its onset) and do not influence established sleep.[8] Prolonged bed rest can have a sinister effect on sleep. Lying flat unleashes thoughts (hence the analyst's couch). Psychological issues often declare themselves in the quiet of night, when visitors have gone home and tiredness encourages reflection and regression. Anxieties and fears during the night, however, present a psychotherapeutic opportunity for the 'night nurse'. The fear, sometimes the hope, of dying in sleep is prevalent, as is the concern that awakening won't happen the following morning. These concerns are real for those experiencing dyspnoea. Physiologically, respiration slows with sleep, as the central drive in response to carbon dioxide stimulation is muted, further compromising oxygenation. Total sleep deprivation is less disturbing than partial deprivation, and actually enhances mood. As an antidepressant therapy it is very difficult to enforce for more than a few nights. Sleep rebound consecutive to sleep deprivation produces an analgesic effect similar to that of paracetamol or a NSAID.[2] Fitful sleep occurs in the anxious. The restless legs syndrome (RLS) may affect 10% of those over 65 years. Precipitated by rest, and relieved by activity, the discomfort is often described as a crawling and tingling sensation in the calf or thigh. The most severe symptoms tend to occur between midnight and 1 am. 'Jumpy' legs responds well to dopaminergic agents; however both opioids and benzodiazepines may help. In palliative care RLS is often serendipitously treated. The periodic limb movement syndrome (PLMS), a rapid stereotypic flexing of the legs associated with repeated awakenings from stage 2 sleep, may be associated with uraemia, neurological diseases, tricyclic antidepressants and stimulants. REM-sleep behaviour disorders (RSB) may occur in neurodegenerative disorders. Pontine damage results in a failure of skeletal muscle inhibition during sleep, so dreams are able to be enacted. The primary treatment is clonazepam, sometimes a medication regime already established. Palliative care patients are at risk of sleep-disordered breathing conditions. Obstructive sleep apnoea occurs more frequently with age and obesity (induced by corticosteroids). Snoring may be noted by others, daytime drowsiness is often the presenting symptom. Central-acting medications are likely to enhance the propensity of apnoea. Awaking hundreds of times during the night severely destroys the recuperative functions of sleep. Early morning awakening (terminal insomnia) may be habitual. It can also be a symptom of a major depressive episode.

The management of insomnia is directed by the aetiology. Improved sleep hygiene, relaxation, symptom relief, supportive psychotherapy, short-term hypnotics, and antidepressant medication are some of the possible interventions. Cheerfulness is discordant with usual feelings of bedtime, and negative thoughts may actually promote the initiation of sleep. Long-term hypnotics cause reductions in stage 3 and 4, the most restful period of sleep, so much sleep is spent in stage 2. Tolerance occurs within weeks, thus efficacy tends to be lost (except for parasomnic symptoms). Methylphenidate, which reduces daytime naps, may improve nocturnal sleep.[9] Melatonin (0.5–6 mg nocte) has both phase-shifting and sleep-promoting properties. It is difficult to anticipate response or determine at what time melatonin should be administered. Thalidomide was initially marketed as a hypnotic, and this effect can be a bonus when used as chemotherapy. Alternative medicines such as valerian, kava kava and chamomile may be effective.

Hypersomnia (drowsiness)

There is a normal circadian propensity to feel sleepy in the early to mid-afternoon. In the general population, 11% of women and 6.7% of men reported daytime sleepiness most days.[10] Drowsiness, mental blunting or torpidity (a mild reduction in alertness) may be disease related, symptomatic of early delirium, or a consequence of medicinal over-sedation. Dissociative type disorders of consciousness are not usually encountered in palliative care practice. Disease burden and fatigue cause excessive daytime sleep. Cerebral injury and degenerative disorders usually cause hypersomnia (and REM behavioural disorders) rather than insomnia. The fatigue associated with CNS damage is profound, accounting for excessive sleep. Returning to infantile sleeping patterns can occur in the twilight of life. Hypersomnia is a symptom of atypical (hibernatory) depression. Sedative adverse effects of medications are potentially correctable, and should be considered in all such clinical situations. Tricyclic antidepressants, anti-emetics (cyclizine, metoclopramide), antipsychotics (levomepromazine), benzodiazepines and opioids can all have residual daytime effects. SSRIs occasionally are associated with daytime sleepiness, perhaps in part because of insufficient sleep. A few escape the worries of life by sleeping (and requesting sedation) and withdrawing (often an indication of depression). Excess sleep, more than 10 h in normal persons, can be associated with the 'blah' syndrome, which consists of tiredness, lethargy and difficulties in thinking and getting going in the morning.[11] Oversleeping does not refresh.

Phase disturbance

Deep sleep by day and interrupted sleep by night is a pattern frequently encountered with involvement of the CNS in the disease. Brainstem sequelae of cerebral haemorrhage and trauma can result in states of prolonged wakefulness. Acute mania needs to be excluded in these patients. Delayed sleep phase syndrome (DSPS), a circadian rhythm disorder, has a familial propensity, is typical of adolescence and is occasionally seen in palliative care settings. Delirium, cerebral metastases, and advanced dementia may be associated with a reversal of the sleep–wake cycle. This syndrome is particularly disruptive to institutional living and notoriously difficult to correct. Bright light modulates the synthesis and release of melatonin, and depending on the time of exposure, light can either phase advance or delay circadian sleep rhythms. Melatonin is most active at the nadir of temperature (about 4 am). With light therapy and melatonin, response rates are about 50%.[12] Attempting to phase shift in a palliative care setting is unrealistic. Sedating medications tend to fade after only a few nights of response as the biological cycle reasserts dominance.

Parasomnia

Parasomnias are not uncommon in palliative care, particularly in those with early CNS disease involvement. Medications increasing stage 3–4 of sleep, such as antipsychotics, can increase the frequency of parasomnia in susceptible persons. Sleep paralysis may occur when falling off to sleep and awakening. There is a dissonance between the level of alertness and muscle atonia. It may be associated with hypnagogic (at sleep onset) and hypnopompic hallucinations (on awaking). Sleep paralysis, if not previously experienced can be terrifying. Sleep walking (somnambulism) can rarely cause accidental injury. Sleeptalking (somniloquy) occurs in stage 1, and despite the fears of the patient, it is generally difficult to comprehend and very seldom, or never, are important aspects of emotional life revealed. Night terrors (pavor incubus) tend to occur early into the night during stage 4 non-REM sleep, and result in waking frightened and aroused with some recall of the content of the dreaming. Benzodiazepines block stage 3–4, are very effective treatments for night terrors, and do not therapeutically fade. Reactivation of PTSD symptoms, particularly night terrors, may occur during severe and life-threatening illness. Hypnic jerks or startle movements falling asleep are common and harmless.

Dreaming

Dreaming occurs mostly during REM sleep. If woken during this phase, recall of the dream is easier. Rehearsal of the dream content immediately upon waking can prevent mentation rapidly slipping from the memory. Dreaming rehearses and reworks events of the day and the entire life in an attempt to find solutions to concerns or predicaments encountered. It allows 'cerebral practising' of actions prior to executing the particular action. Nightmares (or frightening dreams) occur more frequently towards the end of the night, and may provoke wakening. Many psychotropic medications suppress REM sleep (*see* Table 8.1), which probably does not assist psychological adaptation and adjustment. Suppression of REM sleep causes nightmares, possibly due to increased REM intensity over shorter periods.[7] Nightmares are particularly associated with drug withdrawal states (and REM rebound).

Twilight states

Stupor and persistent vegetative state (PVS)

Between alertness and coma are a variety of altered states of consciousness. Stupor is a state of unresponsiveness from which the patient may be aroused by vigorous and repeated stimuli. In palliative medicine it is usually a condition that progresses to coma. The moments of lightened awareness lessen, and responsiveness fades. PVS after severe brain injury consists of wakefulness without awareness. The eyes open spontaneously in response to verbal stimuli, the sleep–wake cycle exists and autonomic functions are maintained. No motor or comprehensible verbal output is possible. The minimal conscious state refers to a similar clinical state in which some semblance of response occurs. Slow visual tracking gives the appearance of communicating, though this is not able to be sustained. In the locked-in syndrome, consciousness is preserved but there is an almost complete inability to respond, only eye movements and blinking being preserved.

Family distress is profound. Visits and care are incredibly arduous. The relatives are relieved that the patient has survived, uncertain how impaired the comprehension and communication really is, and dismayed by the existence of their loved one. Most family members overestimate the retained communication abilities. Intuitive forms of communication occur between family members, but the misinterpretation of reflexive movements as communication is likely. There is often a significant discordance between staff and family about the quality of retained communication. This may have implications for care and its continuance. PVS tends to clinically plateau at about 6 months, but indications of the extent of permanent impairments are not usually offered until after 12 months have elapsed. Until this time the optimism of the family is understandable. Over time (several years often), families visit less frequently and for briefer periods, as reality bites and lives proceed. This is not generally because of fading affections, but rather the necessities of their lives. Issues concerning guardianship, advance directives and site of ongoing care need to be gradually addressed within a supportive family therapy model. With good nursing and medical care these patients may survive years, even decades.

Lightening before death

> We have all observed the mind clear in an extraordinary manner in the last hours of life … we have seen it become capable of exercising a subtle judgement.

Halford wrote in 1842 this clinical description of 'lightening up before death'.[13] This phenomenon is occasionally noted in palliative care units (particularly by nursing staff), however this may be less frequent in modern practice because of the increased use of sedatives.[14] It is often associated with delirium, it is a mortal sign and its occurrence seems impossible to predict. Reduced need for analgesic medications and the short burst of increased vitality immediately before death has been reported, and probably refers to the same clinical event.[15] Hughlings Jackson's theoretical understanding of CNS functioning may account for this phenomenon (*see* Chapter 7).[16] When it does occur it is a wonderful occasion.

Near-death experiences

The literature on near-death experiences (NDE) is generally outside, rather than within, medical publications. Described since antiquity there are some consistent and universal features. Apparently dying, or near to death, enhanced perception to light and cognitive powers occurs. There are varying reports of types and intensity of lights. Enhanced speed and clarity of thought and memory, positive emotions and a belief in having left the body and seeing it from above are the typical symptom clusters in NDEs.[17] The theories proposed to account for this phenomenon are transcendental, psychological and physiological (and combinations of these). Hypoxia must be a component of the cause. Hughlings Jackson's concept of hierarchical dissolution of the damaged nervous system and compensatory positive symptoms would appear consistent with the experiences detailed. Psychological reactions following surviving the near-fatal event must influence how the experience is recalled and processed.[18] Mystical and religious interpretations are likely to be also relevant. The mortality associated with palliative medicine would limit the frequency of such a phenomenon occurring. The relationship of NDE and 'lightening before death' may be that they are variants of the same process.

Last words

It is reported that 30% of patients are alert until moments before death.[19] The very high incidence rates of terminal delirium, coma and medicinal sedation preceding death may suggest this figure is generous.[20] A more recent observation reported only 8% awake just prior to death.[21] Notable actual death bed speeches are probably rare. 'Kiss me Hardy'-type exclamations may be, more commonly than not, mythological. A quoted medical informant in 1961 claimed to have attended 500 deaths without having heard a single memorable utterance.[22] In the ancient world, before death had been medicalised, such events are described and documented. Some Buddhist traditions hope for full lucidity and awareness at the moment of death as an important component of a satisfactory reincarnation.[23] The Roman Catholic last rite provides a final opportunity to be forgiven for sins committed, and presumes clarity and presence of mind. In its endeavour to relieve the suffering of dying, palliative care may also be altering some of nature's kind tricks.

Terminal restlessness

'Terminal restlessness' is a term commonly used to refer to unsettled behaviours during the last few days of life. Consistent clinical descriptions and valid diagnostic criteria are lacking. Terminal anguish, terminal agitation, terminal delirium, agitated delirium and pre-death restlessness are other descriptors of this state. The symptoms include irritability, anxiety, worry, unease, anguish, inattention, hallucinations and paranoia.[19,24–26] The physical signs include restlessness, fidgeting, purposeless yet co-ordinated movements, tossing and turning, trying to get out of bed, moaning, crying out, grimacing, jerking, myoclonus, confusion, picking at the sheets, cognitive impairment and aggression.[24,25,27] The essential features are motor restlessness, emotional distress and delirium.[28] Attempts to develop an objective observer-rated instrument to measure terminal restlessness have not been successful.[26] The prevalence rate during the last 48 h of life is reported to be 42%.[29]

Terminal restlessness is a pseudo-diagnostic term, used predominantly by nursing staff, referring to several conditions causing this array of symptoms and signs. The primary differential diagnoses include poorly controlled pain or discomfort, delirium, medication-induced akathisia, and psychological distress. The reported foci of the psychological distress are the fear of (impending) death, anguish about the life lived, and spiritual issues.[30] Fears of losing control, letting go and the actual process of death are reported themes, as are such issues as 'unfinished business', guilt and 'skeletons in the cupboard'.[19] The initial clinical task is to establish the primary diagnosis. Delirium management differs from managing the fears of dying. In practice, anxiolytic and sedative medication may be resorted to rather too promptly.

Terminal sedation

> Death and his brother Sleep.
>
> Percy Bysshe Shelley (1792–1822)[31]

Death from malignant disease is not always the calm, dignified process so often portrayed on stage and screen.[32] The last 48 h of life may be difficult for 36%, and death 'non-peaceful' for 8.5%.[29] Victorian physicians recorded the invariably peaceful deaths of patients,[33] perhaps in part due to the liberal use of opioids at that time. It may be that modern oncological practice, which has the ability to prolong the life of some cancer patients, is elongating and complicating dying. Sustained and aggressive treatment of the primary malignancy increases the prospects of eventual multi-organ complications. Most patients with cancer do die with comfort and dignity due to the combination of natural processes and medicinal palliation. A minority suffer grave symptoms that defy the skills of multidisciplinary palliative care interventions. Some patients develop intolerable suffering despite excellent care.[34] Intractable symptomatic distress may require deep sedation in order to achieve relief. This practice is referred to as terminal sedation, palliative sedation or sedation of intractable distress of the dying (SIDD). Critics use the terms 'slow euthanasia' and 'backdoor euthanasia'.

Terminal sedation refers to the intentional clinical practice of suppressing consciousness to control refractory symptoms during the last days or hours of life.[35] The intractable symptoms, which have proven non-responsive to all other interventions, are contained by the induction and the continuance of deep sedation. When there is no other medical means of relieving an unendurable symptom, sedation may be the humane clinical option. Intolerable suffering is a medical emergency. It is morally reprehensible to leave a dying patient to suffer intolerably, if there remains a medical option that may ease the suffering. It is crucial to ensure that the symptom is relieved by the sedation, rather than sedating the patient merely to the depth that they are unable to report or communicate their distress. Deep sedation may need to be maintained until death; the duration is usually in the range of 1–6 days.[32]

The intent of sedation is to 'kill' the symptom, and not the patient. Terminal sedation is not 'past cure, past care' (Michael Drayton 1563–1631).[36] The popular presumption is that sedation hastens the end of life. A WHO definition of palliative care incorporates the phrase 'neither hastening nor postponing death'. Deep sedation does not result in a quicker death.[37,38] Deep sedation for terminally ill cancer patients prolongs life.[39,40] The dose of opioid and its rate of increase do not influence survival.[39] The relief of symptoms afforded by the sedation presumably allows greater physiological and psychological comfort while awaiting nature's determination of the time of death. Good nursing care to prevent decubitus ulceration and aspiration is essential. Other life-prolonging interventions have generally at this stage been withdrawn. Terminal sedation may place additional stress on the tired and grieving relatives, by now accepting of the inevitability of the impending death. It also allows an opportunity for the attending family to pause and regroup before the actuality of the death.

Terminal sedation is not physician-assisted euthanasia (PAE). The intent of PAE is to kill the patient (and by this process the intractable symptom). The method is to choose a lethal dose of a medication, rather than a dose that needs to be titrated depending on response. PAE is not a medical intervention.[41] Legal decisions in both the UK and the USA precisely differentiate terminal sedation and PAE on these grounds.[31] The Doctrine of Double Effect discriminates terminal sedation and PAE in terms of the intention to kill. This venerable Roman Catholic principle, originally attributable to Thomas Aquinas, a thirteenth century Dominican theologian, and formulated in relation to self-defence,[42] is internationally accepted as a sound ethical basis for this clinical predicament. According to this doctrine (*see* Box 8.1), if the intent is to achieve a good effect,

---

Box 8.1   The Doctrine of Double Effect (Thomas Aquinas)[41]

An action with two or more possible effects, including at least one possible good effect and others that are bad, is morally permissible if four provisos are met:

- the action must not be immoral in itself
- the action must be undertaken with the intention of achieving only the good effect. Possible bad effect may be foreseen but must not be intended
- the action must not achieve the good effect by means of the bad effect
- the action must be undertaken for a proportionally grave reason (Rule of Proportionality).

---

though the possibility of a bad effect is foreseen, the practice is ethically reasonable.[41] This principle is a doctor-centred concept, with no reference to the patient's world-view. The doctor alone decides intent. Occasionally this scenario can be discussed with patients early in the course of disease, but in reality, and in an emergency, the doctor's interpretation tends to prevail. The Doctrine of Double Effect, however, may not be essential for justification to terminally sedate, as opioids and sedatives have not been shown to abbreviate the last hours of life.[39]

A growing world literature over the last decade reveals that, in palliative care settings, terminal sedation is practised with about 25% of dying patients.[43–45] This does not include the use of medications, usually low-dosage benzodiazepines, to relieve anxiety and/or induce a night's sleep. The first published estimate of the prevalence of the clinical need to terminally sedate, 52.5%, was in a home care programme.[46] Some of the variability of incidence may be related to the type of palliative care facility,[38] though cultural and individual practitioner characteristics also influence. The commonest indication is that of irreversible delirium, a most distressing syndrome for patient, family and staff alike. Profound dyspnoea, uncontrolled nausea and vomiting, acute haemorrhage and intractable pain are other indications (*see* Box 8.2). Opioids are not always available in many countries, and it may be that in these circumstances terminal sedation is more freely practised. Sophisticated analgesic interventions such as nerve blocks, intrathecal delivery systems and surgical procedures, if available, provide alternatives to sedation. Occasionally these techniques also prove ineffective. Surveys,

---

Box 8.2   Terminal sedation: indications

- Irreversible delirium
- Profound dyspnoea
- Intractable pain
- Refractory nausea/vomiting
- Acute haemorrhage
- ? Emotional anguish

---

particularly those from Southern Europe and Asia, indicate that psychological distress or anguish is considered an indication for terminal sedation. The determination of refractory existential distress is complex and deserving of consideration if appropriate and intensive psychosocial interventions have been tried and have failed.[47]

If the possibility of intractable symptoms emerging is discussed with the patient prior to the deterioration of their health status, the clinical decision-making is made more straightforward. This is unlikely. Reassurances of the effectiveness of analgesia are more commonly professed by health professions in the earlier stages of disease. Palliative medicine advertises itself positively. The sufferer of the disease trusts and hopes that reasonable clinical control will be maintained. Anticipating a clinical course is fraught with error. It would be burdensome and inappropriate to discuss these last-resort options.[34] Some patients request that if deterioration causes distress then they would prefer sedation. Anecdotally those persons whom have resorted to 'sedating' the crises in their lives by the use of alcohol, illicit drugs or fierce denial are less prepared to live through dying, and may request sedation. The desire to live fluctuates wildly during a terminal illness, and requests for pharmacological oblivion probably do the same. A request for sleep and sedation may not be accompanied by a wish to die, but merely a desire to have some 'time out' from the intolerable suffering. As the medical crisis is developing, there is often an opportunity to discuss desperate interventions. Consent can often be obtained. The viewpoint of the relatives and proxy are very much more difficult to interpret, and likely to be what they would prefer if they were in that medical predicament.[48] Observing as a bystander is rather different from playing the game. The considerable emotive pressure some relatives place upon medical staff should always be dismissed. If the patient's symptoms can't be controlled by other means, sedation may be considered. A collegial second opinion is a luxury, if available and if time permits. The family needs to be well informed and involved in the decision making. However, CNS involvement of disease may lead to the patient's perception of quality of life being dissimilar to that of carers and others (*see* Chapter 10).

The method of terminal sedation demands pharmacological knowledge and skill. The primary intention is to sedate (to settle, immobilise, induce sleep), rather than to tranquillise or anaesthetise. Benzodiazepines are the medication of choice. They are effective sedatives at higher dose, well tolerated, safe, and versatile with regard to form and route of administration. An antidote (flumazenil) is available. Midazolam is preferred as it is short acting, easy to titrate and compatible with most medications (oral and parenteral) used at the end of life. Concerns regarding anterograde amnestic action are not relevant in this situation. The half-life is extended in the elderly and in those in chronic renal failure. Benzodiazepines can induce confusion at sub-sedative doses. Solid and adequate dosing is necessary. Trial releases of deep sedation can be orchestrated, if required, by withholding the dose or administering flumazenil. The dosage necessary to induce deep sedation is variable. Subcutaneous midazolam 30–60 mg/24 h SC is the usual range. In those with a history of alcohol or substance use (medicinally or illicitly), the required dose may be considerably greater. Theoretically, adding itraconozole or ketoconazole would prolong the half-life, but often at this stage oral compliance is no longer possible. Clinical anecdote suggests that at about 150–200 mg/24 h SC the GABA receptors are fully occupied, or tolerance has occurred, and alternative

---

> **Box 8.3 Clinical questions: sedation and intractable symptoms at the end of life**
>
> - Is this a medical emergency?
> - What does patient (and family) wish for/consent to?
> - What is the quality of (remaining) life of patient (and relatives)?
> - What are the risks and benefits of intervention?
> - What are the ethical and legal considerations?
> - Are there other options/opinions we have not considered?
> - Is the symptom intractable or are the carers 'stumped'?

sedatives need to be considered.[49,50] Age, sex, liver disease and the genetic influences on metabolism account for an up to 10-fold variability in dosing of benzodiazepines. Opioids alone are ineffective sedatives. Phenothiazine medications, such as levomepromazine, can augment the benzodiazepine with its sedating adverse effect. Barbiturates have a narrow safety range and cause centrally induced cardiac and respiratory depression. Chlormethiazole and choral hydrate are difficult to obtain. Propofol, the anaesthetic agent, has been used to induce terminal sedation, but requires considerable skill and anaesthetist expertise. Good documentation and clinical transparency are necessary (*see* Box 8.3). This aspect of practice remains controversial.

Coma

Physical care of the skin and preventing aspiration are essential during this phase. The major focus of psychosocial care shifts from the patient to the relatives. Concerns about whether or not presence or conversations can be appreciated or comprehended are much to the fore. Explanation that Cheyne Stokes respiration is not distressing for the patient, despite the awful auditory discomfort it creates for the relatives, is helpful. Waiting for the inevitable death, sometimes with apprehension, sometimes with impatience, is a vigil for the family. The duration is difficult to estimate. The disease characteristics, including the involvement of the CNS in the disease, and the previous level of cardiorespiratory fitness of the patient may influence longevity at this stage.

The therapeutic intent at this stage should be to assist the relatives cope, relieve their helplessness, and foster good family time. Teaching willing family members to assist with, or assume, some of the nursing duties is very beneficial. It fosters physical expressions of affection, and aborts the sense of passive waiting. It serves as pragmatic family psychotherapy. However some individuals and families find such physical chores abhorrent and too difficult. A not uncommon reason for a terminal admission to a hospice is this. Each family has different attributes and skills in such crises, and these should be identified and therapeutically exploited.

Diagnosing dying

In modern medicine technically disguised dying is commonplace.[51] Doctors and the general public commonly share this illusion, particularly in acute care settings. Futile interventions may be pursued with little expectation of success. Partly this is self-protective for the patient, relatives and doctors. It allows for procrastination and avoidance of contemplating and discussing impending death. Patients often have a sense of impending doom. They know their physiology best. There is no validated, consistently accurate and generally accepted clinical model for predicting life expectancy in cancer and life-threatening illnesses.[51] The medical propensity is to over-estimate survival time.[52] Clinical experience and brief clinical association with the patient (but not a single assessment) improves prognostic accuracy.[52] Clinical judgement plays a significant part, as do various physiological and functional parameters. Ancient Greek physicians considered offering prognoses a crucial component of the profession. While acknowledging their task was easier, as they only had the natural history to consider, the general public demands that modern medicine should be able to do better. The sicker the patient, the more confident can be the prognosis. The history over the preceding hours and days is a guide. The 'road to death' can lead slowly through delirium to coma, or precipitously descend. The 'death rattle', cyanosis, mottling and coolness of the skin and periphery, a cold or white nose, lower limb oedema, a weak pulse, anuria (or sudden polyuria), restlessness and delirium (and coma) indicate that death is likely within hours.[21] Intrusive physical examination is neither appropriate nor instructive. Clinical observation, visually and with olfaction, is usually sufficient. Hippocrates described the characteristic death facies and observed that partial ptosis during sleep or coma was a mortal sign.[53] Eyelid closure prompts sleep (by ensuring darkness), but depends on co-ordinated activity of the brainstem and cranial nerves.[54] A failing brain fails in this task, and bilateral partial ptosis indicates this. Pupillary signs are unreliable in the dying. Opioids cause miosis, but this is an all-or-nothing sign. An ipsilateral Babinski sign is more accurate than pupillary or fundal signs of raised intracranial pressure. Clinicians should be able to discuss frankly the predicament with the patient and attending family if they so wish, adding the proviso that the precise timing of death is not within medicine's jurisdiction allows for the unexpected.

Witnessing dying can be a profoundly disturbing event for some relatives, and a privilege for others. The death of the patient in palliative care signals the commencement of bereavement care. The diagnosis of dying not only ensures sensitive and sensible clinical practice, it introduces this second clinical task of palliative care.

References

1 Paré A. Quoted by FH Garrison in *Bulletin of the New York Academy of Medicine*. 1928; 4: 992.
2 Onen SH, Onen F, Courpron P *et al*. How pain and analgesics disturb sleep. *Clin J Pain*. 2005; 21: 422–31.
3 Moore P and Dimsdale JE. Opioids, sleep, and cancer-related fatigue. *Med Hypotheses*. 2002; 58: 77–82.
4 Cohen MJM, Menefee LA, Doghramji K *et al*. Sleep in chronic pain: problems and treatments. *Int Rev Psychiatry*. 2000; 12: 115–26.
5 Gallup Organisation for the National Sleep Foundation. *Sleep in America Survey*. Princeton: Gallup Organization for the National Sleep Foundation; 1995.

6   De Simone GG. Palliation of pancreatic cancer. *Progr Palliat Care*. 1994; 2: 126–31.
7   Bourne R and Mills GH. Sleep disruption in critically ill patients – pharmacological considerations. *Anaesthesia*. 2004; 59: 374–84.
8   Arnulf I, Boisteanu D, Whitelaw WA *et al*. Chronic hiccups and sleep. *Sleep*. 1996; 19: 227–31.
9   Morita T, Otani H, Tsunoda J *et al*. Successful palliation of hypoactive delirium due to multi-organ failure by oral methylphenidate. *Support Care Cancer*. 2000; 8: 134–7.
10 Hublin C, Kaprio J, Partinen M *et al*. Daytime sleepiness in an adult Finnish population. *J Intern Med*. 1996; 239: 417–23.
11 Globus GG. A syndrome associated with sleeping late. *Psychosom Med*. 1969; 31: 528.
12 Regestein QR and Monk TH. delayed sleep phase syndrome: a review of its clinical aspects. *Am J Psychiatry*. 1995; 152: 602–8.
13 Halford H. *Essays and Orations Read and Delivered at the Royal College of Physicians* (3e). 12 mo, London; 1842, p. 17.
14 Macleod AD and Chaturvedi S. Personal communication.
15 Witzel L. Behaviour of the dying patient. *BMJ*. 1975; 2: 81–2.
16 Dewhurst K. *Hughlings Jackson on Psychiatry*. Oxford: Sandford; 1982, pp. 33–6.
17 Owens JE, Cook EW and Stevenson I. Features of 'near-death experience' in relation to whether or not patients were near death. *Lancet*. 1990; 336: 1175–7.
18 Greyson B. The psychodynamics of near-death experiences. *J Nerv Ment Dis*. 1983; 171: 376–81.
19 Twycross R and Lichter I. The terminal phase. In: Doyle D, Hanks G and MacDonald N (eds). *Oxford Textbook of Palliative Medicine*. Oxford: Oxford University Press; 1993, pp. 658–9.
20 Maddocks I. Last words (Editorial). *Progr Palliat Care*. 2003; 11: 313–14.
21 Morita T, Ichiki T, Tsunoda J *et al*. A prospective study on the dying process in terminally ill cancer patients. *Am J Hosp Palliat Care*. 1998; 15: 217–222.
22 Dennis N. Arthur from the barge. *Encounter*. 1961; 98: 27–31.
23 Maddocks I, Brew B, Waddy H and Williams I. *Palliative Neurology*. Cambridge: Cambridge University Press; 2006, p. 218.
24 Kuebler KK. *Hospice and Palliative Care Clinical Practice Protocol: terminal restlessness*. Pittsburgh: Hospice and Palliative Nurses Association; 1997.
25 Burke AL. Palliative care: an update on 'terminal restlessness'. *Med J Aust*. 1997; 166: 39–41.
26 Jones CL, King MB, Speck P *et al*. Development of an instrument to measure terminal restlessness. *Palliat Med*. 1998; 12: 99–104.
27 Gatera JA, Charles BG, Williams GM *et al*. A retrospective study of risk factors of akathisia in terminally ill patients. *J Pain Symptom Manage*. 1994; 9: 454–61.
28 Macleod AD, Vella-Brincat J and Topp M. Terminal restlessness – is it a fair clinical concept? *Eur J Palliat Care*. 2004; 11: 188–9.
29 Lichter I and Hunt E. The last 48 hours of life. *J Palliat Care*. 1990; 6: 7–15.
30 Rousseau P. Spirituality and the dying patient. *J Clin Oncol*. 2000; 2000–2.
31 Shelley PB. The Daemon of the World: a Fragment, 1815. Pt.1, l.2. *The Complete Poetic Works of Percy Bysshe Shelley*. N Rogers (ed). Vol. II. Oxford: Oxford University Press; 1975, p. 21.
32 Hardy J. Sedation in terminally ill patients. *Lancet*. 2000; 356: 1866–7.
33 Munk W. *Euthanasia: or, medical treatment in aid of an easy death*. London: Longmans, Green and Co.; 1887.
34 Quill TE and Byock IR. Responding to intractable terminal suffering: the role of terminal sedation and voluntary refusal of food and fluids. *Ann Intern Med*. 2000; 132: 408–14.

35 Cherny NI and Portenoy RK. Sedation in the management of refractory symptoms: guidelines for evaluation and treatment. *J Palliat Care.* 1994; 10: 31–8.

36 Drayton M. Richard the Second to Queene Isabel. *Englands Heroicall Epistles.* In: MB Strauss (ed). *Familiar Medical Quotations.* Boston: Little, Brown and Company; 1968, p. 237.

37 Stone P, Phillips C, Spruyt O, *et al.* A comparison of the use of sedatives in a hospital support team and in a hospice. *Palliat Med.* 1997; 11: 140–4.

38 Morita T, Tsunoda J, Inoue S, et al. Effects of high dose opioids and sedatives on survival in terminally ill cancer patients. *J Pain Symptom Manage.* 2001; 21: 282–9.

39 Sykes NK and Thorns A. The use of opioids and sedatives at the end of life. *Lancet Oncology.* 2003; 4: 312–18.

40 Good PD, Ravenscroft PJ and Cavenagh J. Effect of opioids and sedatives on survival in an Australian inpatient palliative care population. *Intern Med J.* 2005; 35: 512–17.

41 Krakauer EC, Penson RT, Truog RD *et al.* Sedation for intractable distress of a dying patient: acute palliative care and the Principle of Double Effect. *Oncologist.* 2000; 5: 53–62.

42 Dunphy K. Sedation and the smoking gun: Double Effect on trial. *Progress in Palliative Care.* 1998; 6: 209–12.

43 Chater S, Viola R, Paterson J et al. Sedation for intractable distress in the dying: a survey of experts. *Palliat Med.* 1998; 12: 255–69.

44 Fainsinger RL, Waller A, Bercovici M *et al.* A multicentre international study of sedation for uncontrolled symptoms in terminally ill patients. *Palliat Med.* 2000; 14: 257–65.

45 Porta Salas J. Sedation and terminal care. *Eur J Palliat Care.* 2001; 8: 97–100.

46 Ventafridda V, Ripamonti C, De Conno F *et al.* Symptom prevalence and control during cancer patients' last days of life. *J Palliat Care.* 1990; 6: 7–11.

47 Morita T, Tsunoda J, Inoue S *et al.* Terminal sedation for existential distress. *Am J Hosp Palliat Care.* 2000; 17: 189–95.

48 Bernat JL. Informed consent. In: Voltz R, Bernat JL, Borasio GD *et al.* (eds). *Palliative Care in Neurology.* Oxford: Oxford University Press; 2004, pp. 387–8.

49 Burns AM, Shelly MP and Park GR. The use of sedative agents in critically ill patients. *Drugs.* 1992; 43: 507–15.

50 Morita T, Tei Y and Inoue S. Correlation of the dose of midazolam for symptom control with administration periods: the possibility of tolerance. *J Pain Symptom Manage.* 2003; 25: 369–75.

51 Dunn GP and Milch RA. Is this a bad day, or one of the last days? How to recognise and respond to approaching demise. *J Am Coll Surg.* 2002; 195: 879–87.

52 Christakis NA and Lamont WB. Extent and determinants of error in doctor's prognosis in terminally ill patients: prospective cohort study. *BMJ.* 2000; 320: 469–73.

53 Hippocrates. *Prognostic.* II.110–118, 6. Quoted in: J Longrigg. *Greek Medicine: from the Heroic to the Hellenistic Age: A source book.* London: Duckworth; 1998, p. 137.

54 Glazer JS. *Neuro-ophthalmology* (2e). Philadelphia: JB Lippincott; 1990, pp. 46–51.

Chapter 9

Neoplasms

[Brain tumours begin with an] imperceptible decline in delicate intellectual processes and a loss of inner emotions.

Hughlings Jackson (1835–1911)[1]

The common tumours within the nervous system, gliomas and cerebral metastases, are rarely curable.[2] The most common primary brain tumour is glioblastoma multiforme. Most high-grade (III or IV) gliomas are terminal within 1–2 years. Brain tumours account for about 3% of cancer deaths. Though relatively unusual, because of their typically long course, brain tumour cases are familiar in palliative care settings. Nervous system metastases are ten times more commonly seen. Cerebral metastases occur in 15–40% of patients with cancer.[3] Lung tumours, melanomas and breast cancers commonly metastasise to the brain, but any cancer may. The prevalence of cerebral metastases is increasing as a result of overall improved survival in cancer patients.[4] Metastatic involvement of cancer tends to be a late complication, the exceptions being lung cancer and melanoma. The majority of metastases occur within the cerebral hemispheres (mainly parietal), and on detection are likely to be multiple (*see* Box 9.1). They can involve the leptomeninges, the spinal cord, the brachial and lumbosacral plexus and the peripheral nerves. Even small lesions can have disastrous effects on quality of life. The natural history of untreated cerebral metastases is progressive neurological deterioration with a median life expectancy of 1 month.[5] Older age, poor performance status and the presence of extracranial metastases are poor prognostic factors.[5] Post-mortem studies suggest up to 30% of cancer patients die with such disease spread, of whom only 50% were symptomatic during life.[6] Sixty per cent of those with small-cell lung cancer, and 75% with metastatic melanoma have demonstrable metastases at autopsy.[3]

The terminal management of malignant tumours affecting the nervous system is challenging. The journey from acute presentation to death can be agonising. Evaluating the benefit–risk ratio in the management of neoplasms is critically important. Avoiding useless 'over-treatment' should be the governing idea.[7]

Symptoms of brain tumours

Headache

Headache occurs at presentation in 36–50% of brain tumours, and during the course of illness in 60% (but in only 40% of those with single metastases). The 'classic' early-morning headache associated with brain tumours only occurs in a minority.[2] Presumably the headache is caused by traction on pain-sensitive brain structures such as the meninges and blood vessels.[2] Early in the course of

---

Box 9.1 Characteristics of brain metastases (adapted from reference 4)

Peak incidence
- 55–65 years

Most common tumour types (adults)
- Lung: 35–45%
- Melanoma: 10%
- Breast: 10–20%
- Colorectal: 5–10%
- Renal cell: 5–10%

Site
- Cerebral hemisphere: 80%
- Cerebellum: 15% (renal, colon)
- Leptomeninges: 8% (breast, lung)
- Brainstem: 5%

Distribution
- Multiple: 70% (melanoma, lung)
- Single: 30% (colon, breast, renal)

Presentation
- Headache: 53%
- Focal weakness: 40%
- Mental/behavioural disturbance: 31%
- Seizure: 15% (melanoma)
- Ataxia: 20%
- Aphasia: 10%
- Asymptomatic: 30%

---

illness the headache may clinically be indistinguishable from tension or vascular headache. Assuming it is psychogenic is usually incorrect in these patients. Though these patients are encountering multiple psychosocial stressors, the headaches are likely to be predominantly 'organic'. If the patient is unable to communicate their symptoms, as may occur in the later stages, observable behavioural signs of pain such as rubbing their head, frowning, shifting restlessly, moaning and groaning suggest the need for improved analgesia. Relatives are often aware of the patient's idiosyncratic or habitual expressions of discomfort, and this can be most helpful to the clinician. If clinical doubt persists, erring on the side of ensuring adequate analgesia is preferable. Severe headache is a most unpleasant pain. A severe headache on awakening (aggravated by coughing or straining), nausea and vomiting, transient loss of vision with papilloedema, sixth nerve lateral rectus palsy, ipsilateral pyramidal limb signs and a deteriorating level of consciousness are suggestion of 'coning' and impending death. Papilloedema is present in only 25% of brain metastases and may be absent even when intracranial pressure (ICP) is very high.

Seizures

Only about 50% of cerebral tumour patients have seizures during the course of their illness.[2] As a presenting symptom, seizures occur in 20–40%. Seizures occur in up to 25% of patients with brain metastases.[3] Seizure prophylaxis is not necessary in those who have never had a seizure, and postoperatively, anticonvulsants may be withdrawn after a week. Prophylactic anticonvulsants are not effective in preventing first-onset seizures in patients with cerebral metastases. Not only do anticonvulsants have cognitive side-effects, they may cause drowsiness, ataxia and hepatotoxicity. There appears to be an increased incidence of severe allergic skin reactions, such as Stevens–Johnson's syndrome, in those patients who have received cranial irradiation and are on anticonvulsants.[8] However the risk of seizures is ever-present and a further source of anxiety for patient and caregivers. In the terminal phase, though a seizure is a rare cause of death, the risks increase as tumour bulk increases. In dying primary brain tumour patients, seizures were a symptomatic concern in only 10%.[9] Oral compliance may not be possible. Benzodiazepines are not particularly effective anticonvulsants in the presence of structural lesions, however they have the advantage of route versatility and do provide a semblance of anticonvulsant cover. Buccal midazolam is the route of choice for status epilepticus in the community. In the hospice, parenteral midazolam would be the likely first choice. There is no demonstrable difference in anticonvulsant efficacy of the various benzodiazepines.

Cognitive dysfunction

Language, visuospatial, memory, and executive dysfunctions may present, depending upon the site and size of the tumour. Radiotherapy, chemotherapy, medications (anticonvulsant, corticosteroid, opioids), post-ictal delirium and depression may all contribute to cognitive deficits. Some may be transient though the already impaired brain becomes increasingly sensitive to insult and less able to recover. Cognitive dysfunction is an important determinant of health-related quality of life and deserves rigorous assessment and, if possible, intervention. Formal psychometric evaluation is time consuming and expensive, and is rarely justified in the terminal phase. Bedside assessment is usually adequate to determine the presence of cognitive impairment and monitor progression over time. The decline of cognitive functioning in brain tumour patients is usually insidious and subtle. The early cognitive deficits may be focal. Rapid change suggests an acute on chronic event such as haemorrhage into the tumour or medication toxicity. Competency issues may emerge as clinical concerns. Management is dependent on the cause of the decline. Adjusting anticonvulsant dosages, altering the corticosteroid regime or treating depression can result in improvement. A trial of methylphenidate has been shown to be of benefit.[10] But inevitably there is a predictable deteriorating course as the mind of the patient is robbed by the neoplasm.

Personality and behavioural change

Subtle coarsening of personality accompanies progressive organic disease of the brain. Mostly the personality changes are minor, sometimes only detectable to close family. Social graces are lost, the usual consideration of others is forgotten, focus becomes more egocentric, and uncharacteristic irritability becomes apparent. Relatives comment that it is as if the patient is very tired after a hard day or late night. The little niceties of the patient's character are lost. There is generally an enhancement of premorbid personality traits. The acquired and practised refinements of adapting to the rigors and reality of life wilt under the burden of organic pathology. The 'organism' reverts to basic self-preservation behaviours. The nervous system regresses to a simpler level of functioning in order to persevere with existence.

Management is to accept these changes, and to manipulate the repertoire if possible. Commonly staff interpret the alterations in behaviour as 'attention seeking, demanding or manipulation'. Forceful, sometimes punitive, reaction and appeals to the patient prove unhelpful. If confronted with interpersonal and cognitive demands beyond their ability to now cope with, catastrophic reactions can be induced. This 'organic motor panic' reaction consists of a transient freezing of motor function and an associated state of anxious perplexity. This extreme response to being cognitively overwhelmed is less common than the hesitant, slowed and measured attempts to respond, which are hopefully recognised by others as indicative of an inability to manage the challenge. By limiting new demands and by encouraging routine these challenges are reduced and behaviours mellow. The same daily routine of ablutions, feeding, resting, accepting visitors and so forth is preferable. Patience, persistence and gentle guidance by staff and relatives should result in the task being eventually achieved. Attending these patients is one of the most demanding of any nursing tasks. The need to correctly pace the patient, intuitively coerce them at times, massage their esteem and sometimes ginger them along are caring skills rarely found, and unfortunately not well appreciated. Obviously to find these attributes in the relatives is chance indeed. Respite care breaks for relatives, who are simultaneously grieving the losses they observe and feel, are essential. Many families cope remarkably well despite the exhausting job. Institutional care, if it is available, is occasionally the most humane option.

Medications have little role. Low-dose benzodiazepine may settle the patient. The use of antipsychotic medication to ameliorate temper outbursts and reduce aggressive behaviour is occasionally of benefit, though there is no evidence to support its use, and the possible neurological side-effects are of concern. Quetiapine has the least potential to cause neurological adverse reactions. The evidence is lacking for anticonvulsant medications for irritable aggression. Buspirone, a novel anxiolytic agent, can rarely and unpredictably be beneficial in these patients. Generally, psychotropic medication for organic personality and behaviour problems is disappointing, and adverse effects are liable to be problematic because of enhanced sensitivity.

Anxiety and mood changes

The propensity to develop sustained and troublesome anxiety, often precipitated by situations, is enhanced in those with brain tumours. The situation with depression is similar, the risk being enhanced by the multiple losses accumulated during the illness. Anxious irritability, rather than overt misery of mood, is not unusual in organic conditions. Both anxiety and depression are more likely early in the course of illness when insight and judgement is retained and the devastating impact on life is able to be acknowledged. Sustained elation of mood is rare.

Assertive multimodal interventions are indicated: individual and family supportive psychotherapy, support groups and medications if appropriate. Being aware of enhanced sensitivity to the adverse reactions of medication should encourage commencing low dosages and gradually titrating to a therapeutic dosage. Response rates are not particularly impressive, perhaps 40–50% in organic mood disorders. The rate of depression in carers is increased, and their welfare should not be neglected.

Hallucinations

Hallucinations may occur. They are usually visual and a part of an epileptic disturbance.[11]

Fatigue

Injury or damage to the nervous system causes profound fatigue. Because the brain has to function at increased capacity to compensate, it tires easily. Within hours of awaking many patients feel physically and emotionally exhausted. Frequent periods of rest need to be programmed, and do help to some extent. When tired, emotions easily become negative and irritable. Fatigue is easily misdiagnosed as depression. Psychostimulants warrant a trial. It is important to withdraw any potentially sedating medications or medications prone to enhance fatigue.

Immobility

Eventually mobility is lost for most brain tumour patients. Specific lesion sites will cause particular losses (e.g. hemiplegia). Steroid-induced proximal myopathy exacerbates mobility problems. Dependency on others is the consequence, and for most losing physical independence is a bitter loss. Immobility heralds the procession of disabling and life-threatening complications including decubitus ulcers, venous thromboembolism, painful contractures and infection. Physiotherapy to maintain and optimise retained function is warranted both from a physical and a psychological perspective.[12] Physiotherapists are reluctant, but very effective, supportive psychotherapists.

Leptomeningeal metastases

Metastases to the leptomeninges are diagnosed in about 5% of those with solid tumours and 50% of haematological malignancies. They occur late in the course of disease.[2] They are frequently missed in the late and terminal stage of illness. Lung, breast, melanoma and lymphomas are the most likely associated maligancies. Multiple neurological losses such as cranial palsies, peripheral nerve lesions, cauda equina lesions, seizures and focal neurological deficits are the typical clinical features.[2] A diffuse, sheet-like covering of the surface of the brain eventuates, and the symptoms may mimic meningitis. It may account for a delirium or cause communicating hydrocephalus.[2] Treatment is generally not contemplated during the terminal phase of illness, other than analgesia if pain is a feature.

Spinal cord metastases

There are few palliative care emergencies. Spinal cord compression is one. This devastating complication is not preventable, but paraplegia may be by prompt intervention. Corticosteroids acutely and immediate radiotherapy are the mainstays of treatment. Very high-dosage dexamethasone, 16 mg to 100 mg IV, can however also result in acute psychiatric side-effects. Delirium, agitation, insomnia, mania and depression can be precipitated and compound treatment co-operation and compliance. The psychological impact of quadriplegia or paraplegia is profound, and the care needs of the patient escalate.

Neuropsychiatric paraneoplastic syndromes

These rare encephalomyelitic syndromes are infrequently recognised by clinicians. They occur in 1% of all cancers and 3% of lung cancers. They may present before the primary tumour. Limbic encephalitis is important in palliative medicine, as delirium is the major differential diagnosis. The typical presentation is a subacute onset of amnesia (mainly short-term), seizures and psychiatric symptoms. These include anxiety, mood lability, confusion, personality change, hallucinations and paranoid delusions. Invariably, denial of the deficits and confabulation cloud the presentation. Most develop progressive generalised neurological signs and dementia. Small-cell lung cancer is the malignancy most often associated. It is a presumed autoimmune response. The course is unpredictable, but generally it stabilises. Treatment of the primary tumour rarely encourages any remission if the CNS is involved. High-dose corticosteroids are advised, but tend to be unrewarding. Residual significant neuropsychiatric disability is the usual outcome. Brainstem encephalitis, cerebellar degeneration, peripheral neuropathy and myopathy may be paraneoplastic.

Psychiatric symptoms and cerebral tumour location

Not only do symptoms change during the evolution of the tumours, the relationship between anatomy and clinical symptoms is relatively imprecise. The compensatory mechanisms of the CNS to adjust to focal lesions are extraordinary. Frontal lobe tumours are typically associated with marked executive dysfunction and personality change, disinhibition or apathy in 90%.[13] Temporal lobe lesions are associated with seizures, often psychomotor in character, and depression. Schizophrenia-like symptoms may be convulsive in origin in these patients. Non-dominant temporal tumours may cause affective syndromes. Parietal tumours rarely produce psychological changes though the dysphasic, dyspraxic symptoms can be mistaken for conversion syndromes or dementia. Occipital tumours are very rarely correlated with mental changes. Corpus callosal tumours are highly correlated with cognitive difficulties. Diencephalic tumours can present with amnestic difficulties including an inability to fixate current events and confabulation, with retained remote memory and other cognitive functions.[11]

The effect on the family

The often long and gradual decline in health and apparent quality of life is stressful for all. 'Social death' occurring months or years before biological death robs the family of the person 'they know'.[14] The loss of 'personhood', competency, appearance and vitality are cruel. Changes in family roles occur as communication is impaired, marital and parental relationships dissolve, finances evaporate and the sheer physical burden of care becomes tiring. The emotional impact upon the family is immense. Faiths and beliefs are challenged by the tragedy. There is, as expected, a wide range of opinion among relatives regarding the trade-off between length of life (and active treatments) and quality of life.[15] Minimal suffering and distress, lack of psychological and cognitive changes, and time spent free of disability, are the outcomes appreciated by relatives, but difficult for the clinician to predict.[15] Support is deserved. Most helpful is information about the disease and treatment, advising the need and right of respite or institutional care, and guiding what is a complex anticipatory grief process. The reality of the predicament is often overwhelming. At the death-bed, family coping difficulties were reported in 85% of families.[9]

Treatment complications

Corticosteroids

The therapeutic benefits of corticosteroids in cancer care are important and at times dramatic. Corticosteroids will produce clinical improvement in 60–70% of those with cerebral metastases, usually within 6–24 h following the initial dose, with maximal effect in 3–6 days.[3,4] Those with symptoms reflecting generalised cerebral dysfunction and raised intracranial pressure from oedema respond more frequently than those with focal neurological symptoms. Corticosteroids double median survival of these patients to two months. The unwanted side-effects can be unpleasant, disfiguring, and disabling. In neoplastic disease longer-term use is generally required and dose and adverse effect profile become major management issues. The appropriate dose of corticosteroid to reduce oedema surrounding tumours is uncertain. A solitary controlled trial concluded that 4 mg, 8 mg and 16 mg of dexamethasone were equivalent over a four-week period, though obviously adverse reactions increased with higher dosage.[16] It is clinical convention to attack with a large dosage, often 16 mg, and then tail the dose slowly towards the lowest possible therapeutic dose. Dose and duration of therapy are important influences upon the adverse effect burden. Psychiatric detrimental effects of steroids occur in 25% and are severe in 5.7%.[17,18]

Psychiatric side-effects

Endogenous and exogenous corticosteroids may affect mood, though 'steroid psychosis' is a misnomer. The rate of depression in Cushing's syndrome is reported to be 50–81%, and mania 27–31%.[19,20] Mood normalises after the cortisol returns to normal. 'Stress' induces glucocorticoid release. In major depressive disorder, hypersecretion of cortisol occurs. The effects on the brain of cortisol vary. In acute and dangerous situations, it prepares the body and mind for 'fight or flight'. If sustained, high cortisol has negative effects on functional activity of the brain, specifically a loss of control of mood (from an evolutionary perspective, a resignation).[19] The mechanisms of acute and chronic steroid side-effects are likely to be different. The acute effects are from a direct upregulation action on the glucocorticoid receptors of noradrenergic and serotonergic neurotransmitters, and/or a normalisation of the hypothalamic–pituitary–adrenal (HPA) axis (by negative feedback).[19] The chronic effects may be due to neurotoxic actions of the glucocorticoids on the hippocampus, reducing glucocortisol receptor plasticity and causing 'steroid resistance'.[19–21] Steroids are poorly absorbed by the brain. High dosage and several weeks of use may be required to induce these changes. Of patients with psychiatric reactions, 77% are on doses greater than 40 mg prednisone.[22] The literature on 'steroid psychosis', from the initial paper in 1952 until currently, consistently describes two syndromes induced by corticosteroids.[23] These are a rapid-onset mild enhancement of mood and wellbeing, tending to fade over a few weeks, and a slower-evolving fluctuating mood disorder, often associated with psychotic symptoms.[22] These problems are commoner in women, at least in the non-cancer literature. However diseases requiring steroid therapy are more prevalent in women and these diseases themselves are prone to psychiatric complications (e.g. systemic lupus erythematosus (SLE)).

Corticosteroid euphoria

This is frequently observed in palliative medicine. Terminally ill patients are prescribed steroids for many non-specific symptoms such as fatigue, anorexia and 'low mood'. The indication to boost/improve mood with steroids was applied to 22% and 12% of hospice patients.[24,25] Improvement of mood in similar patients occurred in 40%, 59% and 71%, though it tended to fade over several weeks.[25–27] The early studies proposed that the euphoria was secondary to improved physical wellbeing.[23] However, in asthmatic patients, mood elevations, but not mania, occurred before the improvement of respiratory function (within a week) in response to approximately 40 mg of prednisone, and settled promptly with discontinuation.[28] There is a suggestion that depressed patients are more likely to get such a response.[28] A modest dose (3–4 mg/day dexamethasone) for 4 days has been shown to improve mood and augment antidepressant action in patients with major depression.[29,30] Response rates of 37% and 60% respectively were noted. Dose does not appear to be relevant in the initiation of this reaction.[22] Insomnia and anxiety induced by steroids may merely be an effect of the physical and mental stimulation of steroids. Corticosteroid euphoria may be induced rapidly in physically compromised 'low-spirited' patients. The benefits seem to fade over several weeks and subsequently the risks of harmful effects of this therapy would seem to increase.

Steroid-induced bipolarity

Mania is the best known, or most memorable, psychiatric adverse effect of steroids. Of the serious psychiatric effects 75% involved mood disorder.[22] Actually depression may be commoner.[17] Mania is reported to occur in 10%, 22% and 40%.[17,31,32] Depression has been reported in 32%.[17] The predominant features of the mood disturbances associated with steroids are rapid fluctuations, mixed mood states and bipolarity.[20] Suicides have been reported.[18] The onset of severe effects appears to take at least a week to emerge, if not longer.[20,32] The clinical similarities of these cases to bipolar disorder are 'striking',[20] as they are to postpartum mood disorder. Psychotic symptoms, described in 11%, occurred as a feature of mania in 40%.[17,32] The descriptions of steroid-induced delirium occurring in 8–25% may be accounted for by this, or by the reality that most of these patients also have severe other medical illnesses.[17,22] Mood disruption is unpredictable, with a possibility of multiple episodes lowering the threshold for future episodes.[22] There is no clear indication that a past psychiatric history increases the risk.[17,22] A report of tricyclic antidepressants aggravating the condition suggests the possibility of an induction of rapid cycling mood fluctuations by steroids.[33]

Steroid dementia

Cognitive deficits have been reported, specifically reversible memory impairment of declarative (verbal) type, suggesting hippocampal involvement.[17,34] There is a case report of six cases of slow resolving 'dementia' on long-term steroids,[35] and another of a single patient.[18]

Steroid dependence

There is a reluctance to cease steroids in palliative medicine practice.[26] There are case reports of psychological dependence, referring to depressive symptoms surfacing on withdrawal.[17,22,36] This may be secondary to the release of the suppression of the HPA axis.[17] Physiological dependence is of course a prominent clinical issue. Abrupt cessation after more than a week of therapy can result in adrenal insufficiency, hypotension and death. In palliative care, discontinuation can be mistakenly implicated as the cause of terminal deterioration,[24] and it has been suggested that this increases terminal restlessness.[25] Fatigue, malaise, anorexia, pyrexia, discouragement, myalgia and arthralgia (pseudo-rheumatism) are anecdotally reported following reduction and withdrawal of steroids.

Body image

Moon facies and weight gain induced by steroids are psychologically disappointing, particularly for women.

Management

Tapering the dose and the administration of psychotropic medications for symptom relief are the two major options. The combination is more effective than these treatments individually.[18] Response within a few days and full recovery is usually expected.[18,20,33] Mania takes longer to settle than depression and delirium, as is to be expected.[22] Drug interactions with anticonvulsants and ketoconazole need to be recognised. TCAs may induce hypomania. SSRIs are probably less likely to do so, but antidepressants should only be used cautiously. Haloperidol is the most commonly used antipsychotic. There are reports of olanzapine and risperidone being used.[22] Lithium carbonate prophylaxis is useful in preventing psychiatric effects of pulse steroids in multiple sclerosis, but has no role in palliative care.

Radiation therapy

The longer survival of cancer patients is demonstrating that the longer-term neuropsychiatric complications of nervous system irradiation can be most disabling. Cranial irradiation increases survival of those with cerebral metastases from 1 month to 4–6 months.[37] Response rate in terms of neurological improvement in cerebral metastases is approximately 50%, and even better relief with other symptoms (headache, nausea) is achieved.[4] Clinically differentiating the effects of radiotherapy from those of the primary illness and other treatments can be difficult.

Radiotherapy to the nervous system results in initial amplification of symptoms because of secondary local oedema. Drowsiness, headache, nausea and a worsening of pre-existing focal symptoms result.[38] Corticosteroids can minimise these. The beneficial effect may take at least 10 days following the completion of radiotherapy to declare itself. Subacute encephalopathy typically presents 1–6 months following completion of radiotherapy. Headache, somnolence, fatigue and deterioration of pre-existing deficits occur secondary to diffuse demyelination.[38] This is spontaneously reversible over several months. Late delayed consequences may appear after 6 months, and these are irreversible and often progressive.[38] Damage to white matter causes symptoms ranging from mild lassitude and minor cognitive slowing to a severe dementia. The prevalence of these complications is uncertain, perhaps a few per cent. Dose and dose scheduling, concurrent chemotherapy and older age are risk factors for these complications. The risks with focal and stereotactic radiation are negligible.

Management options are very limited. Corticosteroids, anticoagulation (to improve microvascular circulation), psychostimulants and occasional surgical excision of a necrosed area are a few potential management options. The tragedy of iatrogenic complications is obvious, and in these cases a very high cost of the prolongation of life.

Chemotherapy

Chemotherapy has an underestimated role in treating patients with brain metastases. Death for half of these patients is caused by the systemic disease, and this treatment may influence survival.[3] The blood–brain barrier is largely destroyed by brain metastases, and drug efficacy is related to tumour sensitivity rather than ability of a drug to cross the barrier. It has been considered that the usually used chemotherapeutic agents do not cause 'chemo-fog'. More careful neurocognitive testing is indicating minor cognitive deficits.[39] Often a good pretreatment cognitive baseline is contaminated by the effects of anxiety, and differentiating disease and treatment consequences is difficult. Lung cancer patients have pretreatment impairments of memory and executive function.[40] Many chemotherapy agents have major acute neurological side-effects including painful peripheral neuropathy (vinca alkaloids), cerebellar ataxia (fluorouracil) and leukoencephalopathy (methotrexate).

References

1 Jackson HJ. Lectures on the diagnosis of tumours of the brain. In: Taylor J (ed). *Selected Writings of John Hughlings Jackson*. Vol 2. New York: Basic Books; 1958, pp. 270–86.

2 Peterson K. Neoplasms. In: Voltz R, Bernat JL, Borasio GD *et al.* (eds). *Palliative Care in Neurology*. Oxford: Oxford University Press; 2004, pp. 37–47.

3 Edwards A and Gerrard G. The management of cerebral metastases. *Eur J Palliat Care*. 1998; 5: 7–11.

4 Lim LC, Rosenthal MA, Maartens N *et al.* Management of brain metastases: review. *Intern Med J*. 2004; 34: 270–8.

5 Gaspar L, Scott C, Rottman M *et al.* Validation of RTOG recursive partitioning analysis classification for brain metastases. *Int J Radiat Oncol Biol Phys*. 2000; 47: 1001–6.

6 Posner JB and Chernik NL. Intracranial metastases from systemic cancer. *Adv Neurol*. 1978; 19: 575–87.

7 Taillibert S, Laigle-Donadey F and Sanson M. Palliative care in patients with primary brain tumours. *Curr Opin Oncol*. 2004; 16: 587–92.

8 Delattre JY, Safai B and Posner JB. Erythema multiforme and Stevens-Johnson syndrome in patients receiving cranial irradiation and phenytoin. *Neurology*. 1989; 38: 194–8.

9 Bausewein C, Hau P, Borasio GD *et al.* How do patients with primary brain tumours die? *Palliat Med*. 2003; 17: 558–9.

10 Meyers CA, Weitzner MA, Valentine AD *et al.* Methylphenidate therapy improves cognition, mood, and function of brain tumour patients. *J Clin Oncol*. 1998; 16: 2522–7.

11 Lishman WA. *Organic Psychiatry: the psychological consequences of cerebral disorder* (3e). Oxford: Blackwell; 1998, pp. 218–36.

12 Huang ME, Cifu DX and Keyser-Marcus L. Functional outcomes in patients with brain tumours after inpatient rehabilitation: comparison with traumatic brain injury. *Am J Phys Med Rehab*. 2000; 79: 327–35.

13 Ron MA. Psychiatric manifestations of frontal lobe tumours. *Br J Psychiatry*. 1989; 155: 735–8.

14 Sweeting H and Gilhooly M. Dementia and the phenomenon of social death. *Sociol Health Illn*. 1997; 19: 93–117.

15 Davies E and Clarke C. Views of bereaved relatives about quality of survival after radiotherapy for malignant cerebral glioma. *J Neurol Neurosurg Psychiatry*. 2005; 76: 555–61.

16 Vecht CJ, Hovestadt A, Verbiest HBC *et al.* Dose–effect relationship of dexamethasone on Karnofsky performance in metastatic brain tumours. *Neurology*. 1994; 44: 675–80.

17 Ismail K and Wessely S. Psychiatric complications of corticosteroid therapy. *Br J Hosp Med*. 1995; 53: 495–9.

18 Lewis DA and Smith RE. Steroid-induced psychiatric syndromes: a report of 14 cases and a review of the literature. *J Affect Disord*. 1983; 5: 319–32.

19 Dinan TG. Glucocorticoids and the genesis of depressive illness: a psychobiological model. *Br J Psychiatry*. 1994; 164: 365–71.

20 Brown ES and Suppes T. Mood symptoms during corticosteroid therapy: a review. *Harvard Rev Psychiatry*. 1998; 5: 239–46.

21 Mitchell A and O'Keane V. Steroids and depression: glucocorticoid steroids affect behaviour and mood (Editorial). *BMJ*. 1998; 316: 244–5.

22 Sirios F. Steroid psychosis: a review. *Gen Hosp Psychiatry*. 2003; 25: 27–33.

23 Rome HP and Braceland FJ. The psychological response to ACTH cortisone, hydrocortisone, and related steroid substances. *Am J Psychiatry*. 1952; 108: 641–51.

24 Gannon C and McNamara P. A retrospective observation of corticosteroid use at the end of life in a hospice. *J Pain Symptom Manage*. 2002; 24: 328–34.

25 Hardy J, Rees E, Ling J *et al*. A prospective survey of the use of dexamethasone on a palliative care unit. *Palliat Med*. 2001; 15: 3–8.

26 Needham PR, Daley AG and Lennard RF. Steroids in advanced cancer: survey of current practice. *BMJ*. 1992: 305: 999.

27 Bruera E, Roca E, Cedaro L *et al*. Action of oral methylprednisone in cancer patients: a prospective randomised double-blind study. *Cancer Treat Rep*. 1985; 69: 751–4.

28 Brown ES, Suppes T, Khan DA *et al*. Mood changes during prednisone bursts in outpatients with asthma. *J Clin Psychopharmacol*. 2002; 22: 55–61.

29 Arana GW, Santos AB, Laraia MT *et al*. Dexamethasone for the treatment of depression: a randomised, placebo-controlled, double-blind trial. *Am J Psychiatry*. 1995; 152: 265–7.

30 Dinan TG, Lavelle E, Cooney J *et al*. Dexamethasone augmentation in treatment-resistant depression. *Acta Psychiatr Scand* 1997; 95: 58–61.

31 Hanks GW, Trueman T and Twycross RG. Corticosteroids in terminal cancer: a prospective of current practice. *Postgrad Med J*. 1983; 59: 702–6.

32 Wada K, Yamada N, Sato T *et al*. Corticosteroid-induced psychotic and mood disorders. *Psychosomatics*. 2001; 42: 461–6.

33 Hall RCW, Popkin MK and Kirkpatrick B. Tricyclic exacerbation of steroid psychosis. *J Nerv Ment Dis*. 1978; 166: 738–42.

34 Wolkowitz OM, Reus UI, Weingartner U *et al*. Cognitive effects of steroids. *Am J Psychiatry*. 1990; 147: 1297–303.

35 Varney NR, Alexander B and MacIndoe JH. Reversible steroid dementia in patients without steroid psychosis. *Am J Psychiatry*. 1994: 141: 369–72.

36 Morgan GH, Boulnois J and Burns-Cox C. Addiction to prednisone. *BMJ*. 1973; 2: 93–4.

37 Patchell R, Tibbs P, Walsh J *et al*. A randomised trial of surgery in the treatment of single metastases to the brain. *N Eng J Med*. 1990; 322: 494–9.

38 Laack NN and Brown PD. Cognitive sequelae of brain radiation in adults. *Semin Oncol*. 2004; 31: 702–13.

39 Anderson-Hanley C, Sherman MI, Riggs R *et al*. Neuropsychological effects of treatments for adults with cancer: a metaanalysis and review of the literature. *J Int Neuropsychol Soc*. 2003; 9: 967–82.

40 Meyers CA, Byrne KS and Komaki R. cognitive deficits in patients with small cell lung cancer before and after chemotherapy. *Lung Cancer*. 1995; 12: 231–5.

Chapter 10

Cognitive dysfunction and dementia

A crust of indifference is slowly creeping around me, a fact I state without complaining. It is a natural development, a way of beginning to grow inorganic; the detachment of old age I think it is called.

Sigmund Freud (1856–1939)[1]

The rapidly rising rates of dementia worldwide, a reflection of aging populations and lifestyle, signal an emerging crisis. 'Too few cradles, too many graves' will be an issue for future generations. Palliative medicine does not attend to patients with dementia. There are a few exceptions.[2] A palliative approach to dementia care and partnership, rather than specialist palliative care, may offer the best benefit to the burgeoning services for the elderly. Patients suffering cancer also may be experiencing age-related cognitive dysfunctions and treatment-related cognitive deficits (*see* Chapter 9). Cognitive failure impacts upon coping with the dying process, sometimes aiding it, mostly not.

Cognition and pain

Older persons tend to be more stoical about pain. Pain is expected and tolerated with advanced age. They complain less, sometimes using words such as 'aching', 'soreness', and 'discomfort' provokes acknowledgement. Patients with cognitive impairments are less likely to receive analgesia, and the risk of under-treatment increases with the severity of dementia.[3,4] In demented patients expressions of pain may be different and difficult to interpret. Analgesics may be over-used or under-used as a consequence. If the patient is able to communicate, self-report rating scales (e.g. visual analogue scales) are used. These target sensory-discriminative aspects of pain, its presence and intensity. If non-communicative, observatory scales are used and these provide information about motivational-affective aspects of pain. Facial expressions are reliable indicators. Pain can affect any behaviour, so it is useful to have a baseline of eating, sleeping and exercising patterns. A change in a behavioural pattern may indicate pain. However no change may not reflect the absence of pain.[3] Atypical responses such as frowning, combativeness, withdrawal, and agitation may signal pain. Guarding, bracing, moaning, fidgeting and muscular tenseness are less indicative of pain and may be symptoms of extrapyramidal dysfunction or other distress. Autonomic responses such as changes in blood pressure and heart rate are not particularly sensitive indicators.[3] Pain thresholds are not different in Alzheimer's dementia (AD), however pain tolerance is significantly increased.[5] The pain stimulus is received but its processing is impaired. The neurological basis for motivational-affective processing is severely affected in AD, whereas the primary sensory areas

Table 10.1 Common procedures and pain (10-point numeric rating scale)[6]

Procedure/experience	Mean pain rating
Nasogastric tube	6.9
Phlebotomy	4.6
Indwelling urethral catheter	4.3
Intramuscular injection	3.9
Mechanical restraints	2.4
Movement (chair to bed)	2.0
Chest radiograph	1.4
Vital signs taken	1.3
Waiting for a procedure	1.1

are not. Pain is felt but experienced with less (different) distress. Observation is more relevant than self-report rating scales in demented patients. Basic medical and nursing procedures are surprisingly uncomfortable (*see* Table 10.1).[6]

Dementia

Dementia is a chronic and progressive clinical syndrome characterised by an acquired impairment of three domains of function: neuropsychological (amnesia, aphasia, apraxia, agnosia, executive dysfunction), behavioural/psychological (or more correctly psychiatric) symptoms (BPSD), and deficits in activities of daily living (ADL) (sufficient to interfere with occupational performance and social interactions). Dementia is distinguished from mental retardation by its acquired nature. Demented persons are at high risk of delirium because of a low deliriant threshold (*see* Chapter 7). Amnestic syndromes and aphasia are more focal impairments. Depressive pseudodementia can mimic dementia, but the history usually provides differentiation. These patients, unlike those with dementia, complain of poor memory and provide 'don't know' (can't be bothered) answers to routine questions. A normal shedding of interest in current world events as terminal illness enters its final phase can be mistaken for the apathy and disinterest of dementia. In benign senile forgetfulness (or mild cognitive impairment), the deficits are predominantly slowing of performance, and are non-progressive. Reversible causes of dementia are rare. The commonest type of dementia is AD (60%) followed by vascular dementia (VD) (20%). Dementia with Lewy bodies (DLB) accounts for 15%, and frontotemporal dementia (FTD) 5% (*see* Table 10.2).

The disease trajectory is slowly progressive. The rate and the pattern of this deterioration depend upon the pathological process. Late-stage dementias are similar, irrespective of the type of disease. Every disease is person-specific, and clinically there is huge variability. The final stage of AD may last a year or so, and for many this is spent in institutional care. This is not usually hospice care. In nursing home care, advanced dementia patients are not perceived as having a terminal condition, and most do not receive optimal palliative care.[11] In a tertiary hospital, 63% of dying demented patients were assessed as having high levels of suffering, 30% intermediate and only 7% had low levels.[12] The majority

Table 10.2   The salient features of the dementias

	History	Mental status	Neurology	Comment
Alzheimer's disease (AD)	Gradual onset	Anterograde amnesia	Subtle if present	Commonest
	Memory and behavioural presentation	Visuospatial deficits		A diagnosis of exclusion
		Apraxia, agnosia, anosognosia		
Vascular dementia (VD)	Abrupt onset	Dependent on regions affected	Focal deficits	Differentiating AD and VD is arbitrary, there is considerable overlap[7]
	History of stroke Stepwise progression	Psychiatric symptoms early		
Dementia with Lewy bodies (DLB)	Cognitive fluctuations	Attention	Extrapyramidal signs	? Identical to the dementia of Parkinson's disease
	Visual hallucinations	Visuospatial deficits		Most responsive to cholinesterase inhibitors (greater cholinergic loss)
	Parkinsonism Antipsychotic sensitivity	Preserved memory		
Frontotemporal dementia (FTD)	Insidious onset	Executive (frontal lobe) signs	? Motor weakness	May evolve bulbar signs and motor neurone disease (MND)[8]
	Loss of personal/social awareness	Memory often normal	Fasciculations	MND may evolve into FTD
	Disinhibition/ impulsivity	Inability to infer mental state of others		Semantic and progressive aphasia not associated with MND
	Loss of judgement			

Table 10.2 (*Continued*)

	History	*Mental status*	*Neurology*	*Comment*
Creutzfeldt–Jakob disease (CJD) (a prion disease)	Rapidly progressive	Perplexed, apathetic mental state	Dysphagia	Sporadic
	Mood lability	Lability of mood	Incontinence	Acquired in 5% (diet, iatrogenic)
	Myoclonus/ seizures	Gross global cognitive deficits	Sensory hypersensitivity	Mood lability, apathy precede neurological symptoms by several months[9]
	Cerebellar/ visual dysfunction		Rigidity	Distressing for relatives and staff[10]
			Dystonia	Fatal within months
			Stupor	
AIDS dementia complex (ADC)	Social withdrawal	Inattention	Ataxia	Symptoms and course influenced by highly active antiretroviral therapy (HAART)
	Apathy	Slowed thinking	Tremor	
	Irritability		Abnormal reflexes	
Huntington's disease	Dysmentia rather than a dementia	Slowing of cognitions	Chorea, athetoid movements	Psychiatric symptoms precede chorea and dementia
	Personality change	Depressed mood	Rigidity	
	Depression	Psychosis	Dystonia	

died 'restless'.[12] There are no disease-modifying treatments available, however deterioration may be delayed by medications such as the cholinesterase inhibitors. Dementia shortens life expectancy. The median survival time from initial diagnosis is 4 years in men and 6 years in women, and less if the age on onset is young.[13] The actual cause of death in these patients is dementia, though the event is commonly 'pneumonia'.

Clinical assessment of advanced dementia

In palliative care settings a diagnosis is generally established prior to referral. Cortical dementia (e.g. AD) presents with prominent memory, language and visuospatial deficits. Subcortical dementia (e.g. AIDS dementia complex (ADC), DLB, Huntington's disease) characteristically have impairments of speed of cognition, executive and mood features, with less prominent amnesia. Easy confirmation of significant organic deficits is by using the Executive Clock Drawing

Test (CLOX) which assesses the visuospatial and visuoconstruction abilities and the executive skills required to set a clock.[14] However it does not differentiate dementia, delirium and opioid intoxication.[15] Neither does the MMSE. A test of category fluency ('name as many animals as possible in one minute', expecting 15 at least in normal individuals) is also a convenient one-minute confirmatory test of advanced dementia.[16]

Management of neuropsychological impairments

Adjustment issues

Individual psychotherapeutic support, because it is difficult and unrewarding, tends not to be persevered with. Acceptance is not mentioned in the eight-stage process individuals are assumed to use to interpret their illness: slipping, suspecting, covering up, revealing, confirming, surviving, disorganisation, decline and death.[17] Encouraging a process of narrative review, of recording life stories, can be affirming and rewarding. The loss of 'personhood' and 'social death' predate death. Caregivers considered that over one-third of demented dependent were socially ('as good as') dead prior to biological death.[18]

Amnesia

Memory can be unlocked by emotions, particularly negative ones.[19] Anger or sadness may unleash memories of trauma. Such memories are more forcefully laid down originally and are more difficult to forget. These memories in turn may unlock surrounding memories, the 'flashbulb' effect. Continuing to challenge cognitive functions preserves them. Education and 'exercising the brain' are protective and lessen the rate of decline.[7] Cholinesterase inhibitors may improve memory in 25% and delay deterioration. Repetition, reassurance, and redirection are necessary, and frustrating, tasks for carers.

Communication

Communication difficulties become increasingly problematic. Receptive impairments (attention, comprehension, agnosia), expressive troubles (apraxia, aphasia, dysarthria) and interpersonal stressors (disinterest, apathy, depression) compound management. Language is eroded, health workers increasingly communicate with the carer and not the patient, and the focus of emotional support shifts towards the caregivers. Providing functional spectacles and hearing aids, and proper dental care should not be neglected.

Advance directives

Living wills or advance directives are infrequently executed and often lacking in specific detail with respect to management of a particular illness. When written, the nature of the terminal disease probably was not known. In emergency situations medical staff are likely to proceed as they deem necessary to save life. Medical circumstances are in a state of continual flux. Living wills are static documents and generally unable to accommodate the dynamic changes of disease and the emotional responses to it. The major attribute of advance directives is that the process involves communication and discussion of the medical issues between patient, family and health professionals. They are based on the concept of respect for autonomy and on the patient's right to self-determination. These egocentric views of individual rights have been challenged in non-Western cultures in which family and community interests may prevail. At some stage during the course of dementia, competency to make personal decisions about possible treatment options is lost. The right of informed consent is transferred to a legally authorised surrogate decision-maker to exercise, on the patient's behalf, healthcare decisions. The surrogate, preferably a close relation, is required to follow the explicit and implicit preferences of the patient. Organising this person early, and discussing with them possible disease and decision scenarios, is very helpful. Surrogacy can be a lonely task.[20] Intrafamily relationships are invariably complex. Empirical studies suggest that substituted judgements are erroneous in approximately one-third of attempts.[21] Particularly when making decisions about end-of-life, the surrogate tends to be conservative and choose life, rather than being the 'executioner'.

Competence

Competence or capacity refers to the making of a particular decision.[22] It refers to a categorical status. 'Decisional abilities' are dimensional and include the ability to understand, appreciate, reason and express choice. This can be reasonably estimated by a series of questions (*see* Box 10.1). Competence is more subjective and is determined by expert opinion rather than objective evaluation. There is a lack of clear criteria. Inter-rater agreement may be poor. Competence involves multiple domains of intellectual functioning. The predominant domain is 'executive' function. Scores below 18 on a MMSE usually indicate incapacity, above 24, capacity. Specific tests of executive function, such as word fluency, are likely to be more accurate.[22] Deciding on a treatment option may be possible in severe dementia, though the patient may not possess testamentary capacity. Decision-making ability may not be decisional competence. A feature of disease to the nervous system is organic denial. As degeneration of the CNS proceeds, the will to live, or the reluctance to appreciate the deterioration of quality of life, strengthens. The patient may come to contest their own advance directive, made when more competent.

Box 10.1   Assessment of decisional ability and competence

1   Why does the issue of competency arise now?
2   Does the patient know what his current circumstances are?
3   Does the patient know what his options are?
4   Does the patient know the consequences of each available choice?
5   What is the patient's reason for making a particular choice?
6   Is the patient consistent in his decision?
7   Is there any undue influence?
8   Can the patient act on or execute the choice made?

Management of behavioural/psychiatric symptoms of dementia

BPSDs are responsible for many of the management problems relating to the care of dementia patients, increased caregiver stress and increased rates of institutionalisation. They occur in up to 80% of patients, usually in the mid- to late stages of disease (*see* Table 10.3).

Agitation

Agitation is common. Anxiety is often expressed as agitation. Agitation refers to inappropriate verbal, vocal, or motor activity that is not judged by an outsider to result directly from the needs or confusion of the patient. It may be a behavioural response to pain, irritation, frustration, over-sedation, boredom, loneliness, sensory over-stimulation, or invasion of personal space and privacy (particularly in the apathetic patient). Attending to the source relieves the clinical sign. Social interactions help reduce the severity of disruptive behaviours.[23] 'Pet therapy' (regular visits or contact with an animal) showed an improvement in irritability.[24] Aromatherapy has been shown to settle agitation.[25] Antipsychotic medications are widely used, particularly if aggression is a problem. There is little convincing evidence of effectiveness of typical antipsychotics. Haloperidol (0.5– 6 mg daily) may reduce aggression but not agitation.[26] Neurological effects, falls and a possible acceleration of cognitive decline are adverse reactions of these drugs. Atypical neuroleptics (risperidone, olanzapine) have a good evidence base for effectiveness in behavioural symptoms,[27] but the threefold increased cardiovascular risk may preclude their use, or at least this needs to be incorporated into the risk–benefit equation.[28] The efficacy of anticonvulsants is suggestive but not conclusive. Cholinesterase inhibitors are possibly helpful.[29] Memantine, a NMDA-receptor antagonist, shows promise. Antidepressants are indicated if affective symptoms contribute. High-dose vitamin E and oestrogens may be of value. Benzodiazepine studies from the 1960s showed benefit, but concerns of disinhibition limit their use (*see* Chapter 2). Placebo responses of 30% suggest that the staff attention shown, and the associated interactions, is modestly therapeutic. Training and support of staff in non-drug management strategies reduces antipsychotic use by 20%.[30]

Table 10.3 Behavioural and psychiatric symptoms of dementia

Psychiatric symptoms	Behavioural symptoms
Depression (up to 80%)	Personality changes (up to 90%)
Delusions (20–73%)	Agitation, restlessness (60%)
Misidentification (23–50%)	Aggression (20–50%)
Anxiety (12–50%)	Catastrophic reactions
Hallucinations (15–49%)	Wandering, shadowing
Mania (3–15%)	Screaming
	Hoarding
	Culturally inappropriate behaviours
	Cursing

Wandering

Aimless walking, attempts to leave the environment (to go home), and shadowing of caregivers are examples of this troublesome and potentially dangerous symptom. Prevalence rates of 50% are reported, usually in the mid-stage of disease. It is often as if the patient stays as physically active as their body allows for they have a sense that soon this ability will be lost forever. This is a major problem in Huntington's disease patients in whom ataxia and falling are additional significant risks. Structured recreational walks can reduce agitation in wanderers.[31] Collusion then redirection is the only management strategy likely to contain this activity. Mild sedation can aggravate wandering.

Catastrophic reactions

Rage reactions, or brief periods of paralysing indecision and perplexity occur if and when cognitive abilities are overwhelmed by external challenges. They may be verbal and/or physical and associated with anxiety and panic. Limiting and pacing cognitive demands reduces the frequency, and anxiolytic medication may diminish the anxious response.

Depression

Depression occurs in at least 40% at some stage. This is often early in the course and may not last even if untreated.[32] Affective symptoms are common, though severe depression is not, and suicidal ideation is reported in only 4%.[33] Mood symptoms tend to peak early in the course of dementia, whereas motivational symptoms (avolition, social and emotional withdrawal) increase with the severity of dementia. There are surprisingly few treatment studies. TCAs are usually not tolerable and SSRIs are preferred. Psychostimulants and cholinesterase inhibitors warrant consideration, and ECT should not be easily dismissed as a treatment option. Response rates, particular in VD, are often only modest.

Anxiety

Anxiety presents as agitation rather than psychic worry. It tends to fade as insight diminishes. Anxiety contaminates psychometric testing. Caregiver anxieties often increase as dementia advances.

Delusions

Misidentification, misplacement and forgetfulness provoke paranoia. Persecutory and paranoid delusions are persistent in 20%. Antipsychotics do improve 20–30% of those experiencing delusions.

Hallucinations

Visual hallucinations are common in DLB and delirium complicating dementia.

Sleep disorder

Insomnia, hypersomnia, delayed sleep phase syndrome and REM behavioural sleep disorders are associated with dementing disorders (*see* Chapter 8). Bright light therapy, similar to the treatment used in seasonal affective disorder, has been shown to improve sleep in demented patients.[25]

Apathy and disinhibition

Frontal lobe dysfunction initially results in loss of behavioural control and aggression. With progression of disease apathy increasingly dominates. Management with behavioural and antipsychotic medications may mute the impulsive responses. Psychostimulants deserve a trial in apathetic patients but there comes a time when the dopamine receptors no longer have the capacity to respond.

Management of deficits of activities of daily living

Occupational difficulties created by the gradual onset of dementia are invariably difficult and distressing for all concerned. Handling money, driving, using the telephone, dressing, feeding and eventually toileting difficulties are the typical array of daily living tasks that become problematic. Safety concerns become relevant – access to smoking materials, medicines and poisons, electrical appliances, dangerous stairs and roads all necessitate supervision and monitoring. Generally there is a long period of disabling symptoms and marginal self-care. The management decisions that are required to be made during the course of dementia are symptomatic of the crisis of modern medicine. That is, because an intervention is technically possible, it must be offered. Nature's decision making ultimately can't be defied by modern medicine, though the journey can be made tortuous by it.

Nutrition

Eating difficulties develop as dementia progresses. Apraxia complicates the mechanical task of eating, co-existent depression destroys appetite, bulbar involvement impairs swallowing, olfaction and taste changes dissuade appetite, and hunger may not be able to be perceived. Hand feeding, antidepressant medication and a fluid diet respectively may assist. There is no evidence that long-term feeding tubes are beneficial in individuals with advanced dementia.[34] They increase the risk of aspiration and they do (partially) deprive the patient of the pleasure of eating and the companionship of sharing food.

Hydration

It is claimed dying of dehydration is not unpleasant and that good mouth care and sips of fluid provide adequate symptom control.[35,36] Severe dehydration may contribute to delirium and this is the most persuasive indication for hypodermoclysis.

Resuscitation

Cardiopulmonary resuscitation (CPR) in demented persons is medically futile. Only 1% of demented residents in a nursing home suffering cardiac arrest can be expected to be discharged alive from hospital.[2] The dilemma for the clinician is that of discussing 'Do not resuscitate' orders. At what stage in the course of dementia does CPR become a futile intervention?

Place of care

New unfamiliar and frightening environments, such as hospitals, and the medical risks of interventions need to be considered and weighed against the potential benefits. Emergency departments and hospitals expose the demented to serious risk.[2] Antibiotic treatment of chest infections neither relieves discomfort nor prolongs survival in advanced dementia.[37]

References

1   Freud S. Letter to Lou Andreas-Salomé, May 10, 1925. Quoted in: Freud E, Freud L, Grubrich-Simitis I (compilers). *Sigmund Freud: his life in pictures and words*. St Lucia: Queensland; 1978, p. 237.
2   Volicer L. Dementias. In: Voltz R, Bernat JL, Borasio GD *et al.* (eds). *Palliative Care in Neurology*. Oxford: Oxford University Press; 2004, pp. 59–67.
3   Scherder EA and Bourma A. Is decreased use of analgesics in Alzheimer's disease due to change in the affective component of pain. *Alzheimer's Dis Assoc Discord*. 1997; 11: 171–4.
4   Scherder E, Oosterman J, Swaab D *et al.* Recent developments in pain and dementia. *BMJ*. 2005; 330: 461–4.
5   Benedetti F, Vighetti S, Ricco C *et al.* Pain threshold and tolerance in Alzheimer's disease. *Pain*. 1999; 80: 377–82.
6   Morrison RS, Ahronheim JC, Morrison GR *et al.* Pain and discomfort associated with common hospital procedures and experiences. *J Pain Symptom Manage*. 1998; 15: 91–101.
7   Snowdon DA, Lernfelt B, Landahl S *et al.* Brain infarction and the clinical expression of Alzheimer's disease: The Nun study. *JAMA*. 1997; 27: 813–17.
8   Hou CE, Carlin D and Miller BL. Non-Alzheimer's disease dementias: anatomic, clinical, and molecular correlates. *Can J Psychiatry*. 2003; 49: 164–71.
9   Spencer MD, Knight RSG and Will RG. First hundred cases of variant Creutzfeldt-Jakob disease: retrospective case note review of early psychiatric and neurological features. *BMJ*. 2002; 324: 1479–82.
10 Bailey B, Aranda S, Quinn K *et al.* Creutzfeldt–Jakob disease: extending palliative care nursing knowledge. *Int J Palliat Nurs*. 2000; 6: 131–9.
11 Mitchell SL, Kiely DK and Hamel MB. Dying with dementia in the nursing home. *Arch Intern Med*. 2004; 164: 321–6.
12 Aminoff BZ and Adunsky A. Dying dementia patients: too much suffering, too little palliation. *Am J Alzheimers Dis Other Demen*. 2004; 19: 243–7.
13 Larson EB, Shadlen MF, Wang L *et al.* Survival after initial diagnosis of Alzheimer's disease. *Ann Intern Med*. 2004; 140: 501–9.
14 Sutherland T, Hill JL, Mellow BA *et al.* Clock drawing in Alzheimer's disease: a novel measure of dementia severity. *J Am Geriatr Soc*. 1989; 37: 719–25.

15 Manos PJ. The utility of the ten-point clock test as a screen for cognitive impairment in General Hospital patients. *Gen Hosp Psychiatry.* 1997; 19: 439–44.

16 Duff Canning SJ, Leach L, Stuss D *et al.* Diagnostic utility of abbreviated fluency measures in Alzheimer's disease and vascular dementia. *Neurology.* 2004; 62: 556–62.

17 Keady J and Nolan M. Younger onset dementia: developing a longitudinal model as a basis for a research agenda and as a guide to interventions with sufferers and carers. *J Adv Nurs.* 1994; 19: 659–69.

18 Sweeting H and Gilhooly M. Dementia and the phenomenon of social death. *Sociol Health Illn.* 1997; 19: 93–117.

19 Williams DDR and Garner J. People with dementia can remember. *Br J Psychiatry.* 1998; 172: 379–80.

20 Bernat JL. Informed consent. In: Voltz R, Bernat JL, Borasio GD *et al.* (eds). *Palliative Care in Neurology.* Oxford: Oxford University Press; 2004, pp. 383–93.

21 Sulmasy DP, Terry PB, Weisman CS *et al.* The accuracy of substituted judgements in patients with terminal diagnoses. *Ann Intern Med.* 1998; 128: 621–9.

22 Kim SYH, Karlawish JHT, Caine ED. Current state of research on decision-making competence of cognitively impaired elderly persons. *Am J Geriatr Psychiatry.* 2002; 10: 151–65.

23 Cohen-Mansfield J and Werner P. Management of verbally disruptive behaviours in nursing home residents. *J Gerontol.* 1997; 52: M369–M377.

24 Zisselman MH, Rovner BW, Shmuely Y *et al.* A pet therapy intervention with geriatric psychiatry inpatients. *Am J Occupl Ther.* 1996; 50: 47–51.

25 Burns A, Byrne J, Ballard C *et al.* Sensory stimulation in dementia: an effective option for managing behavioural problems (editorial). *BMJ.* 2002; 325: 1312–13.

26 Lonergan E. Haloperidol for agitation in dementia (Cochrane review). *The Cochrane Library Issue 2: CD002852.* Oxford: Update Software; 2002.

27 Curran S, Turner D, Musa S *et al.* Psychotropic drug use in older people with mental illness with particular reference to antipsychotics: a systematic study of tolerability and use in different diagnostic groups. *Int J Geriatr Psychiatry.* 2005; 20: 1–6.

28 Keys MA and De Wald C. Clinical perspective on choice of atypical antipsychotics in elderly patients with dementia, Part II. *Ann Long Term Care.* 2005; 13: 30–8.

29 Wynn ZJ and Cummings JL. Cholinesterase inhibitor therapies and neuropsychiatric manifestations of Alzheimer's disease. *Dement Geriatr Cogn Disord.* 2004; 17: 100–8.

30 Fossey J, Ballard C, Juszczak E *et al.* Effect of enhanced psychosocial care on antipsychotic use in nursing home residents with severe dementia: cluster randomised trial. *BMJ.* 2006; 332: 756–61.

31 Aronstein Z, Olsen R and Schulman E. The nursing assistants' use of recreational interventions for behavioural management of residents with Alzheimer's disease. *Am J Alzheimer's Other Demen.* 1996; 11: 26–31.

32 Brodarty H and Luscombe G. Studies on affective symptoms and disorders: depression in persons with dementia. *Int Psychogeriatr.* 1996; 8: 609–22.

33 Draper B, Moore CM and Brodarty H. Suicidal ideation and the 'wish to die' in demented patients: the role of depression. *Age Aging.* 1998; 27: 503–7.

34 Gillick MR. Sounding board rethinking the role of tube feeding in patients with advanced dementia. *N Eng J Med.* 2000; 342: 206–10.

35 Hoefler JM. Making decisions about tube feeding for severely demented patients at the end of life: legal and ethical considerations. *Death Stud.* 2000; 24: 233–54.

36 Twycross R and Lichter I. The terminal phase. In: Doyle D, Hanks GWC and MacDonald N (eds). *Oxford Textbook of Palliative Medicine* (2e). Oxford: Oxford University Press; 1998, p. 500.

37 Hurley AC, Volicer B, Mahony MA *et al*. Palliative fever management in Alzheimer patients: quality plus fiscal responsibility. *Adv Nurs Sci.* 1993; 16: 21–32.

Chapter 11

Terminal neurological disorders

I am not only a skeleton but a badly articulated one to boot. If to this is coupled the fact of the creeping paralysis, you have the complete horror.

WNP Barbellion (1889–1919)[1]

The typical course of these illnesses may be at least one to two decades. Determining the terminal phase can be uncertain. Death is sometimes eventually rather unexpected. The shift from an acute interventional medical model, necessary to preserve quality of life, to allowing a terminal decline is often clinically a passive process. Respiratory, gut and skin problems are undoubted issues in the final phases of these patients' lives, but troublesome neuropsychiatric symptoms present major management challenges. Dying is difficult, dying with an already compromised nervous system is very difficult.

Parkinson's disease

Since the discovery of levodopa in the 1960s the treatment of Parkinson's disease (PD) has been revolutionised.[2] Approximately 10% of PD patients present before the age of 50 years and can live well for 20–30 years with modern treatments. The disease in older onset patients tends to have a less favourable course. Within 5–10 years, problems with drug unresponsiveness, dyskinesias, dementia and depression compound management.[1] The terminal phase may last 1–2 years.[2]

Anxiety and depression

Movement is the fundamental nervous system function. For it to be slowed (bradykinesia) and inefficient is a primal wound to any organism. Anxiety is a consequence. To be frozen in movement is an innate fear. A state of utter helplessness ensues. This brief moment of 'death' may induce unease, panic and even PTSD. In patients with on–off fluctuations, anxiety is more often related to the off phase. Anxiety is higher if mobility is less.[3] Depression may be precipitated during the latter phases of PD, particularly if other risk factors are present. Differentiating psychomotor retardation and bradykinesia is difficult. Depression, probably an integral part of the disease, occurs in more than 40%.[3] Anxiety tends to be a prominent feature of this depression. Depression is commoner in those with more severe cognitive impairments and a past affective history. Apathy and depression may co-exist. Depression is a risk factor for PD, and may be the presenting symptom.[3] Suicide and alcoholism rates in PD are low. SSRIs are the most tolerable antidepressant choice. Tricylics' anticholinergic properties potentiate the risk of delirium but may have a mild anti-parkinsonian action. The response rates in 'organic' depressions are often disappointing. ECT should not be discounted, and it has the added advantage of improving motor symptoms as well as mood.[4]

Dementia

Dementia complicates at least 30% of PD, particularly in the elderly.[3] In the majority, Lewy bodies are present. Bradyphrenia, the slowing of cognitive processes, is a feature. With progression, apathy becomes increasingly evident. Cholinesterase inhibitors warrant a trial.

Psychosis and complications of dopaminergic therapy

Psychosis occurs in approximately 30% and is usually caused by levodopa therapy in younger patients.[3] In the elderly it may indicate the emergence of dementia, which further lowers the threshold to tolerate dopamine agonist therapy. Hallucinations and illusions are mainly visual, occasionally tactile and olfactory. These sensory aberrations are often fleeting. Fluctuating persecutory and paranoid delusions often accompany them. Delirium needs to be excluded and the dose of antiparkinsonian medication reduced if possible. Meticulous drug fine-tuning does not invariably result in easing the adverse effects. Antipsychotic medications risk aggravating the movement disorder. The newer atypical neuroleptics are preferred. Low-dosage quetiapine or olanzapine are usually tolerated with only minimal neurological adverse reactions. The most effective and safest medication is clozapine, though sedation may be problematic. The required doses are generally very low (15–50 mg/day), but there is a risk of blood dyscrasia. Tremor may also be improved with clozapine. Ondansetron has been trialled for this indication, and in dementia cholinesterase inhibitors may be an alternative to antipsychotic medication.[3] Neurosurgery and deep brain stimulation may be indicated, a reflection of the enormity of the distress these medication adverse effects may create. Less distressing and equally embarrassing are the array of motor fluctuations, dyskinesia, akathisia, hyperkinesia, dystonia and chorea that may occur at various dosing intervals. These patients are generally extremely reluctant to reduce their dopamine dose even fractionally, appearing to be addicted to them.[2] Hypersexuality is occasionally a problem. Partners are very unlikely to volunteer this information without prompting. Erectile failure is a more common symptom in PD. Excessive gambling is a possible risk of dopaminergic medications.

Pain

Stiffness and rigidity caused by PD can be uncomfortable.[2] Dystonic and dyskinetic movements can be painful. Antispasmodic medications, local botulinum toxin injections and adjustment of the dopaminergic regime may be indicated. Intermittent apomorphine can be useful.[5] Constipation is inevitably a problem due to poor gut mobility. If opioids are introduced, a laxative regime is necessary. If opioids induce nausea, domperidone is the anti-emetic of choice as it does not cross the blood–brain barrier.

Sleep disturbance

Sleep is fragmented in PD. Dopaminergic medications induce vivid dreams, often precursors to a psychosis. REM behavioural disorders are more frequent. Restless legs at night can be disruptive and painful. It is usually treated with dopamine agonists, however clonazepam and opioids do often provide some respite. Day-time sleepiness is a consequence of the night-time disruptions.

Terminal Parkinson's disease

If there is bulbar involvement, chest infections may be the eventual cause of death. Akinetic rigidity is the usual preterminal motor state. During the terminal phase, oral compliance may be compromised. Apomorphine infusions may be useful at this stage at doses of up to 50 mg/24 h. Pretreatment with domperidone is preferable as nausea is a major adverse effect of apomorphine.[6] The risk of induction of hallucinations is possibly less than with other dopamine agonists. Parenteral anticholineric agents severely aggravate delirium, but are an option if the patient is sedated. Abulia, an impairment of will, or an inability to initiate behaviour and actions (including speech, creating akinetic mutism), is a possible complication of late-stage PD. The phasing out of the dopamine agonists account for this, and apomorphine warrants a trial for this distressing symptom.

Multiple sclerosis

In multiple sclerosis (MS), inflammatory focal demyelination of the nervous system causes a myriad of sensory, motor and neuropsychiatric symptoms. The natural course of the disease is extremely variable. The disease burden accumulates for the majority, and after 2–3 decades a progressive deteriorating course is assumed. Irreversible neurological deficits create physical dependency and psychiatric morbidity.[6] Overall life expectancy is seven years less than normal. Mortality increases with disability. Infection is the most common cause of death.[7] There is no cure for MS. Disease-modifying agents, such as interferons and glatiramer, may influence the natural course. This for most is subtle, and may merely prolong the duration rather than the quality of life.

Psychological adjustment is made most difficult for symptoms wax and wane. They are unpredictable, embarrassing and invisible. They erode physical and psychological autonomy. Fatigue is a core disabling feature. The inevitable march of MS undermines individuals and families.[8] The lifetime prevalence of depression is 40–60% and is related to cerebral involvement of the disease, though this is not clearly correlated with MRI scan lesion load.[6] Disruption of frontal-temporal circuits by plaques may be the critical organic risk factor for depression, as well as for bipolar mood disorders which have a two-fold increased incidence. There are generally a host of psychosocial adversities further enhancing the risk of affective disorder. Suicide rates are elevated 7.5-fold, especially in the young.[6] Interferon medications can induce depression. SSRIs are likely to be the most tolerable antidepressants. Persons with already compromised CNS functioning detest any further loss in function such as that induced by psychotropic medication adverse effects.[8]

Eutonia, euphoria, pathological laughing/crying and lability of mood may respond to cognitive and distracting strategies and low-dose antidepressants.[9] They occur in 10–25% of MS patients, usually in those more severely affected. Cognitive impairments occur in 40–60% and are severe in 21–33%.[6] The dementia is 'subcortical', the deficits being a slowing of cognitive processing, impaired auditory attention, memory retrieval difficulties and executive function impairments. Language and memory are not manifestly impaired. The dementia of MS is easily missed at the bedside, yet hinders daily living significantly. Superimposed depression may amplify these cognitive deficits. The impact on employment, tasks of daily living and competency is considerable. Management options are limited. Recognition allows the possibility of others assisting in compensating for the deficits. Cognitive retraining and memory cues may help in the early stages. If associated with a significant neurological relapse, high-dose corticosteroids may warrant a short course. Cognitive enhancing medications such as the cholinesterase inhibitors have been trialled. Personality change, particularly apathy, irritability and disinhibition, are subtle indicators of the slow organic disintegration of MS, rather than being intentional 'attention-seeking' behaviours.

By the time of death, the person who developed MS decades previously is, sadly, hardly recognisable. Bedbound and cognitively a shadow of their prior self, the patient in the frail terminal physical state may be best humanely not actively treated. MS directly rarely actually causes death.

Stroke

Stroke is a heterogeneous group of diseases which include brain infarction, intracerebral bleeding, subarachnoid haemorrhage and rare entities such as vasculitis and vessel dissections. About 20% die within one month of a stroke, and 10% in the following year, so within 2 years one-third have died.[10] Many deaths are sudden, caused by acute progression of the strokes. Only one-quarter fully recover, and 40–50% experience some form of disability.[11] Stroke units, thrombolysis and lifestyle education may improve prognosis and prevent stroke, but the aging population is likely to increase the rates over subsequent decades. There is an enlarging population of severely disabled, dependent survivors who have psychiatric and palliative needs. Additionally 15% of cancer patients have cerebrovascular lesions at autopsy, and 50% of these lesions might have been symptomatic.[12]

Acute stroke results in 'modified mental processing'.[13] Difficulties with remembering the event and anosognosia (and denial) influence judgement and decision making. Emotional incontinence, sadness, mild disinhibition, catastrophic reactions and anxiety over the first few weeks suggest depression, and may be eased by low-dosage antidepressants. These acute psychological wounds tend to settle over time. Weeks to months later, post-stroke depression may evolve in up to 40%, of which 25% is major depression.[13] Guilt, hopelessness and suicidal ideation tend not to be prominent depressive features. Mood lability and rehabilitation inertia dominate. Co-existent depression amplifies cognitive impairments. The location of the stroke is a minor risk factor for depression compared with severity, functional outcome and cognitive damage.[13] Assertive antidepressant trials are indicated. The earlier literature advocated nortriptyline, however the critical influence to choice is tolerability. Most use SSRIs as first choice. Fatigue (independent of depression) haunts rehabilitation. Psychostimulants can be of benefit, though usually pacing activities and demands is more therapeutically enduring. Stroke patients with limited cerebral reserves are at high risk of delirium. Communication difficulties, particularly with left-sided lesions, are a crucial challenge of management. This is made especially difficult if there is also cognitive impairment (which is highly likely). Memory, spatial awareness and personality may all be affected. Post-stroke dementia occurs in 20–25%. Pain is a prominent problem post-stroke, often within weeks. The 'shoulder-hand syndrome', headache and 'central post-stroke pain' are difficult conditions to treat. Aphasic patients have been shown to receive less analgesia.[14]

The devastating consequences of stroke not only affect the patient. The burden of care on others is immense. The rates of depression in carers are high. Short respite admissions are valuable, and also provide an opportunity to review changing care needs. Bereavement support can easily be instituted at this time, and better prepares both patient and relatives for the uncertain future ahead.

AIDS

HIV-positive status has immense impact on relationships, family, occupation and society. HIV is a potent neurotoxic agent and enters the CNS early in the course of illness. HAART therapy, if available, has radically altered the neuropsychiatric complications. Adjustment issues are liable to be influenced not only by the personal circumstances of the patient but also by the characteristics of the society they live in. Drug abuse, impoverished socioeconomic circumstances, lifestyle and social stigma may be relevant influences. Fatigue is an invariable complaint. Neuropathic pain may complicate in about 30–50%.[15] Pain management in the drug-using HIV-positive patient is challenging (see Chapter 12). Major depressive disorder and the elevated risk of suicide deserve appropriate interventions. Suicide risk may be enhanced by impulsive behaviour and emotional lability, though most suicides occur early in the disease. Acute manic episodes may be indicative of early dementia, as mania is usually associated with cognitive impairments. The abrupt presentation of psychotic symptoms should be clinically considered to be an infective delirium until this has been excluded. Psychosis tends to herald dementia. Subtle personality and cognitive changes may occur early and potentially influence adjustment processes, decision making, and compliance with medications. Interruptions of medication compliance are liable not only to risk progression and complications, but subsequent re-introduction may prove ineffective. Cognitive impairment is present in 20–30% of those who are not on HAART therapy. The advent of HAART and longer survival are factors actually increasing the prevalence of cognitive impairment and AIDS dementia complex (ADC), but perhaps reducing its severity. The incidence of AIDS dementia has halved post-HAART from 7%/year to 3%/year, but the prevalence has doubled because of the increased survival.[15,16] HAART provides only partial protection from the neurotoxicity of HIV. HAART is changing the typical neuropsychological features either directly or by delaying presentation to an older age group and thus adding other risk factors for dementia. ADC is not

Table 11.1 Clinical features of AIDS dementia complex (ADC)

	Early	*Late*
Cognitive	Inattention Poor concentration Forgetfulness Slowed thinking	Global dementia
Motor	Ataxia Impaired handwriting Tremor Urinary urgency/hesitancy Impaired rapid alternating movements Abnormal reflexes Leg weakness	Paraparesis Incontinence
Behavioural	Social withdrawal Apathy Irritability/mania	Mutism

an inevitable consequence of HIV infection and nor is it always progressive.[16] ADC is subcortical dementia with cognitive, motor and behavioural symptoms (*see* Table 11.1). Insight can be preserved until late.[16] Differentiation from depression can be difficult, and therapeutic trials of SSRIs and psychostimulants are not to be dismissed. ADC is a clinical diagnosis and many decline formal neuropsychological evaluation for this merely highlights the deficits and provides no therapeutic advantage. Deficits able to be recognised by the self, such as memory impairment and psychomotor co-ordination, increase the desire for death, whereas executive dysfunction and abstract reasoning difficulties do not.[17]

The profound neurological sensitivity to antipsychotic medications limits use. Clozapine, the most effective of the antipsychotic medications also has the fewest neurological side-effects. Benzodiazepines are well tolerated but sedative at higher dose. Antiviral medications, particularly those that penetrate the CNS and are used in combination, may cause insomnia and depression in less than 10%. Neuroprotective agents such as memantine and seligiline may have a role.

The clinical course of AIDS is erratic and difficult to predict, even with good medication compliance. A major clinical dilemma in the terminal phase is whether or not antiviral and prophylactic antibiotic medications are continued or not. Risking terminal opportunist infection is not necessarily wise, as uncontrolled symptoms such as diarrhoea may cause a very prolonged and uncomfortable death.[18] Very assertive medical care is generally required to protect quality of life, and withdrawing this towards the expected end of life can be problematic. Orchestrating a 'good death' in AIDS patients may not be possible. Early in the course of the epidemic, palliative care institutions were sometimes available for these patients. In countries with access to newer therapies the illness has been transformed into a manageable chronic illness, and the supportive phase may last decades.[18] The mean time from diagnosis to death has increased from 6 months to over 48 months.[16] If accumulated neurocognitive deficits enforce institutional care for the long-term survivors, then palliative medicine's role is likely to be required again. Death in AIDS is often stigmatised.[19] It may be embarrassing to the family and secretive; customary bereavement rituals may not be performed. The burden of shame complicates grieving.

Motor neurone disease

No cure is known for motor neurone disease (MND). It most commonly presents in the sixth decade and has a prognosis of 3–4 years for most, though rarely it may be longer.[20] With the exception of the marginally effective riluzole, no treatment is known. The reactive distress and profound weakness experienced and the sedative adverse effects of antispasticity agents and anxiolytic medications can easily mislead the clinician into thinking that depression is compounding the illness. Pseudobulbar affect (emotional lability and incontinence, pathological laughing/crying) is a feature in about 50%.[21] This can be symptomatic of depression and of dementia. It may be eased by (low-dose) antidepressants. SSRIs tend to be preferred. While tricyclics may beneficially reduce drooling, they may also thicken respiratory secretions and increase tenacity, as well as aggravating constipation. Any clinical hint of depression deserves psychosocial and medication intervention. Communication aids are critical to the quality of remaining life. Assessment of cognitive functioning in MND patients is difficult because of the communication struggles. Clinicians are reluctant to examine cognition for it really just confronts the patient with the recognition of further losses. There is an association between MND and frontotemporal dementia (*see* Chapter 10). MND patients are wary of medications as they are very protective of their remaining function and are reluctant to risk CNS side-effects. Swallowing problems are ultimately inevitable, and assisted feeding and ventilation are issues that require consideration. They are not without beneficial and adverse effects. Pain caused by spasm, cramps and immobility requires physiotherapy and analgesic medication. With advancing weakness and physical dependency, anxiety about the process of death becomes a preoccupying concern for many. Suffocation and 'choking to death' are actually rare.[22] Rapidly progressive respiratory failure is the usual terminal event.

Muscular dystrophy

These predominantly genetic disorders result in early death. The commonest, Duchenne's muscular dystrophy (DMD), is an X-linked recessive trait, occurring predominantly in males, affecting pelvic and pectoral musculature but sparing smooth and bulbar musculature.[23] Death by respiratory failure and infection usually has occurred by the age of 25 years.[23] Mild intellectual impairment has been associated with DMD. Because of difficulties clinically ascertaining cognition and mental status, the neuropsychiatric aspects of these diseases are less well established. The implication of muscle weakness and wasting on an adolescent, the developmental phase most sensitive to body image conflicts and self-esteem doubts, is obviously massive. The family, who experience genetic guilt and anger, tend to focus their care in purely physical ways by concentrating, often exclusively, on signs of progress and (begrudgingly) deterioration. The stress of the family unit is immense. More than one child may be affected. Marital discord is common, divorce being reported in up to 24%.[24] Such high rates of marital disillusion are typical of relationships that suffer child loss. The course of disease is usually about a decade. Management decisions such as those relating to assisted ventilation are not infrequently made during an emergency. Rarely can these individuals and families proactively come to such decisions. Professionally one seems helpless, unable to infiltrate the often very firm defences these families use for protection. Issues of fears of choking, ventilatory panic and relating to ongoing ventilation quandaries (both for patient and carers) are sometimes the first opportunity for palliative and psychosocial interventions. Explanation, reassurance, benzodiazepines for anxiety, and opioids for respiratory distress, may ease the terminal phase.

References

1 Barbellion WNP. *The Journal of a Disappointed Man*. London: The Hogarth Press; 1948, p. 274.
2 Clough CG and Blockley A. Parkinson's disease and related disorders. In: Voltz R, Bernat JL, Borasio GD *et al.* (eds). *Palliative Care in Neurology*. Oxford: Oxford University Press; 2004, pp. 48–58.
3 Nilsson FM. Psychiatric and cognitive disorders in Parkinson's disease. *Curr Opin Psychiatry*. 2004; 17: 197–202.
4 Moellentine C, Rummans T, Ahlskog JE *et al.* Effectiveness of ECT in patients with Parkinsonism. *J Neuropsychiatry Clin Neurosci*. 1998; 10: 187–93.
5 Bowron A. Practical considerations in the use of apomorphine injections. *Neurology*. 2004; 62(suppl 4): S32–S36.
6 McDonald WI and Ron MA. Multiple sclerosis: the disease and its manifestations. *Phil Trans R Soc Lond B*. 1999; 54: 1615–22.
7 Sadovnick AD, Ebers GC, Wilson RW *et al.* Life expectancy in patients attending multiple sclerosis clinics. *Neurology*. 1992; 42: 991–4.
8 Macleod AD and Formaglio F. Demyelinating disease. In: Voltz R, Bernat JL, Borasio GD *et al.* (eds). *Palliative Care in Neurology*. Oxford: Oxford University Press; 2004, pp. 27–36.
9 Feinstein A. *The Clinical Neuropsychiatry of Multiple Sclerosis*. Cambridge: Cambridge University Press; 1999, pp. 65–79.
10 Kwakkel G, Wagenaar RC and Lankhorst GJ. Predicting disability in stroke – a critical review of the literature. *Age Aging*. 1996; 25: 479–89.
11 Hamann GF, Rogers A and Addington-Hall J. Palliative care in stroke. In: Voltz R, Bernat JL, Borasio GD *et al.* (eds). *Palliative Care in Neurology*. Oxford: Oxford University Press; 2004, pp. 13–26.
12 Graus F, Rogers LR and Posner JP. Cerebrovascular complications in patients with cancer. *Medicine*. 1985; 64: 16–35.
13 Bogousslavsky J. Emotions, mood, and behaviour after stroke. *Stroke*. 2003; 34: 1046–50.
14 Kehayia E, Korner-Bitensky N, Singer F *et al.* Differences in pain medication use in stroke patients with aphasia and without aphasia. *Stroke*. 1997; 28: 1867–70.
15 McArthur JC. HIV dementia: an evolving disease. *J Neuroimmunol*. 2004; 157: 3–10.
16 Brew BJ. HAART in AIDS dementia complex and palliative care. *Prog Palliat Care*. 2004; 12: 171–7.

17 Pessin H, Rosenfeld B, Burton L *et al*. The role of cognitive impairment in desire for hastened death: a study of patients with advanced AIDS. *Gen Hosp Psychiatry*. 2003; 25: 194–9.

18 Maddocks I, Brew B, Waddy H and Williams I. Incurable infections of the nervous system. In: *Palliative Neurology*. Cambridge: Cambridge University Press; 2006, pp. 170–7.

19 Chandra PS, Deepthivarma S and Manjula V. Disclosure of HIV infection in south India: patterns, reasons and reactions. *AIDS Care*. 2003; 15: 207–15.

20 Oliver D and GD Borasio. Diseases of motor nerves. In: Voltz R, Bernat JL, Borasio GD *et al*. (eds). *Palliative Care in Neurology*. Oxford: Oxford University Press; 2004, pp. 79–89.

21 Abrahams S, Goldstein LH, Kew JJM *et al*. Frontal lobe dysfunction in amyotrophic lateral sclerosis: a PET study. *Brain*. 1996; 119: 2105–20.

22 Neudert C, Wasner M and Borasio GD. Patients' assessment of quality of life instruments: a randomised study of SIP, SF-36 and SEIQoL-DW in patients with amyotrophic lateral sclerosis. *J Neurol Sci*. 2001; 191: 103–9.

23 Maddocks I and Stern L. Muscular dystrophy and related myopathies. In: Voltz R, Bernat JL, Borasio GD *et al*. (eds). *Palliative Care in Neurology*. Oxford: Oxford University Press; 2004, pp. 90–6.

24 Buchanan D, LaBarbera C, Roelofs B *et al*. Reactions of families to children with Duchennes muscular dystrophy. *Gen Hosp Psychiatry*. 1979; 1: 262–8.

Chapter 12

Chronic mental illness and dying

> I can feel I am dying, and dying quickly ... I was mad and now I am sane.
>
> Cervantes (1547–1616)[1]

Those who suffer chronic psychiatric ill-health can also experience life-threatening and terminal illnesses. When a terminal illness is diagnosed the presumptions of the patient, relatives and carers are often not only that the pre-existing psychiatric illness will be exacerbated, but also that the patient will 'not cope' and the medication regime 'will need to be strengthened'. This is not necessarily correct. Many cope very well; for some their mental condition actually improves, and others struggle desperately.

Affective disorders

The natural history of a depressive episode is for spontaneous resolution. This generally occurs between six months and ten years; however predicting this occurrence is not possible. Antidepressant medications merely palliate the depressive symptoms, until this resolution occurs. Depression recurs in at least 50% of patients. With each recurrence, clinicians tend to maintain antidepressant medication for longer periods, and after more than a few recurrences many are advised to stay on a therapeutic dose of a tolerable and effective medication indefinitely. Terminally ill patients who are taking an existing antidepressant regime should be continued on this regime. The dosage may need to be reduced if renal and hepatic functions deteriorate. Patients with a known history of prior depression who experience a relapse during terminal illness should be recommended on this previously effective antidepressant.

Spontaneous resolution of a depressive episode may occur during the course of a terminal illness. Clinical impression suggests that this occurs not infrequently. Many historical psychiatric treatments involved physiologically and psychologically 'shocking' the patient. Cold douching, violent rotation, fever therapy, and insulin and electrical convulsive therapies are such examples.[2] Freud commented that melancholia may be brought to a temporary end by intercurrent organic disease.[3] There is a number of case reports of such recoveries.[2,4] This phenomenon is also commonly observed in the few days following a suicide attempt. Transiently mood lifts, and occasionally it resolves. It is speculative as to whether the mechanism is psychological or physiological.

Bipolar affective disorders present particular management difficulties in palliative care. High-dosage corticosteroids (above 40 mg equivalent dose of prednisone) can induce mood instability, particularly in those who are predisposed (*see* Chapter 9). This may take weeks to settle even with the cessation of the steroid and antimanic medications. AIDS is particularly associated with mania, and because of sensitivity to the neurological side-effects of antipsychotics, benzodiazepines and mood stabilisers may need to be relied upon in these patients. Lithium carbonate remains the mood stabiliser of first choice for bipolar illness. However it has a narrow therapeutic range, and at toxic levels lithium carbonate is dangerous. Acute delirium and neurological signs (tremor, parkinsonism) are clinical indicators of toxicity. Urgent serum levels must be obtained. Fever, dehydration and renal impairment predispose to lithium toxicity. Ceasing maintenance lithium carbonate is associated with an increased incidence of manic swings several months later. Lithium for many of these patients has been very valuable, and they may be reluctant to cease it. Alternative mood stabilisers such as sodium valproate, carbamazepine and lamotrigine, if tolerable, are not as efficacious, and a terminal illness is not an occasion to trial alternatives. Lithium carbonate should preferably be continued and reviewed very carefully (with frequent serum monitoring). Benzodiazepines do possess antimanic properties, and clonazepam can prove a safe and effective option. There is no literature concerning the impact of a terminal illness upon chronic dysthymia. Anecdotally the distractions of severe physical illness often redirect anxiety and worry onto the patient's oncological status. Adjustment issues and oncological stressors may trigger reactive mood dips. It is as if the ongoing health concerns validate the dysphoria and reinforce mental health invalidism. Generally, antidepressants are prescribed as 'cover', though if therapeutic gains can be made it is usually in response to psychosocial therapies. Unhappy people are likely to die unhappy.

Psychotic disorders

Delay of presentation of physical symptoms resulting in delayed diagnosis is a particular concern in schizophrenia. Hidden fungating breast wounds, ignored rectal bleeding and apparent insensitivity to pain make the detection of underlying malignancy more difficult in these patients, even if they are resident in an institution. The lack of response to the emergence of physical symptoms is multifactorial.[5] Difficulties verbalising the symptoms, extraordinary tolerance of discomfort and pain, fear of disclosure to medical and nursing staff with whom they may have fraught relationships, anxieties about trusting others, the incorporation of the 'new' symptom into their existing delusional system, and the withdrawn negative symptoms of schizophrenia may all contribute.[5,6] For the attending psychiatrist it may be the distraction of focusing upon the primary psychiatric illness, and minimising the physical symptoms, that contributes to delayed recognition. Astute (junior) staff in psychiatric hospitals can and do diagnose cancers and other serious medical illness early.

Management may be made easier for the patient if they have an existing therapeutic relationship with an individual or a system. However if paranoia and trust issues are evident, management may be most difficult and sometimes impossible. The reclusive elderly paraphrenic, the hostile and chaotic young male who complicates a psychotic illness with substance abuse, and the apathetic negativistic catatonic schizophrenic are clinical examples of such patients. Close liaison with family and the attending psychiatric staff is critical. Adjustment of the existing psychotropic regime may be necessary. Some require downward increments of antipsychotic medications, particularly if the cancer has CNS involvement. A minority require higher doses. Irrespective of the particular antipsychotic medication the patient may be maintained on, it is still advisable to use additional haloperidol as first-line medication in delirium (*see* Chapter 7). If the delirium reverses then the haloperidol is able to be withdrawn, and the original antipsychotic regime remains in place.

Institutionalised patients often consider the psychiatric hospital their 'home', and wish to be managed in this familiar environment by nursing staff, whom they know and trust, until death. The oncology ward or the hospice are new situations and perhaps too difficult to contemplate. 'Their own' nursing staff is generally delighted to respond, with palliative care support, to the new challenge of terminal care.

Alcohol dependency

Oblivion is a kind of Annihilation.

Thomas Browne (1605–1682)[7]

Heavy and sustained alcohol use is a risk factor for many malignancies. Many decide not to alter their alcohol consumption after the emergence of a terminal illness. Some reform. All experience, but rarely will discuss, the guilt and the regret of substance- and self-induced disease. Establishing psychotherapeutic relationships at this stage is most difficult. Invariably, many past attempts at therapy and sobriety have failed. Most interpret these failures of therapy as 'not their fault'. They project blame onto many of the well-meaning and competent clinicians involved, rather than acknowledge personal responsibility for harmful and antisocial behaviours. Personality, mental ill-health and circumstances may have led to the excessive reliance on alcohol. Decades of such behaviour and consequent mild brain damage create a rigid and unpsychological style of coping, and making psychotherapeutic gains is resisted. In crises, the coping strategy so commonly used by alcoholics is to use alcohol and induce a state of oblivion. It is not infrequent that such patients in their terminal phase request deep sedation. Because of past alcohol use (and often prior exposure to benzodiazepines) higher sedative dosage than usual may be required. Delirium tremens (DT) should be considered if a sudden alteration of behaviour and consciousness occurs 2–3 days after an admission (*see* Chapter 7). Alcoholic hallucinosis is usually associated with the withdrawal of alcohol use, and less commonly with resumption of use after a dry period. Wernicke's encephalopathy (weakness, peripheral neuropathy, ophthalmoplegia), a thiamine deficiency state, is associated with alcoholism, but can be secondary to malabsorption syndromes and inadequate vitamin supplementation in feeding regimes of cancer patients.

Alcoholics have families, many of whom have been damaged by the patient's lifestyle and a few of whom are co-dependent. Invariably a distressed and disturbed family raises issues for palliative care staff. While these families should not be treated differently from others, they may well deserve the expertise of services other than palliative care. A crisis is a therapeutic opportunity, and irrespective of the past it may be the occasion to forge a different future for the surviving family.

Substance abuse disorders

Substance use is a major risk factor for cancer and AIDS. Smoking and illicit drug use is unhealthy. These facts are public knowledge. How the individual comes to terms with the awareness that these habits are causing their demise depends on the circumstantial and psychological reasons initiating such risky behaviours. Veterans of World War II may hold their respective military services responsible for encouraging and supplying cigarettes. Developmentally traumatised individuals may have been forced into, or found temporary respite in, drug use. There are as many explanations as there are drug-using patients. Drug use in most communities is increasing. The modern control emphasis is on 'harm minimisation' rather than abolition. Influencing mankind's innate interest in mind-altering drugs and stopping illicit supply have proven rather ineffective. Over future decades, more terminally ill persons with substance abuse histories will be attended to in palliative care.

Street drug use by opioid-dependent and addicted cancer patients poses major difficulties in palliative care settings. They may have been expelled from drug maintenance services for the crisis of their physical health persuaded them to abandon the rules of the programme. Having decided that death is now inevitable, risk-taking behaviours may escalate. Careless and fatal miscalculations of street supplies can result, as may admission to general hospitals with acute cellulitis or endocarditis. Doctors' opiophobia may result in pseudoaddiction, the patient seeking additional medication secondary to inadequately managed pain.[8] The terminally ill opioid-dependent cancer patient will require a maintenance dose of opioid plus an analgesic dose (see Box 12.1). Methadone is the usual maintenance opioid in drug programmes because of its long half-life and limited diversion prospects. Buprenorphine and naltrexone are more difficult to supplement with analgesics.[9] Generous dosing regimes are required to achieve pain relief. This may be related to a 'tolerance memory' or more probably to the fact that the underlying personality is poorly practised in, or incapable of, delaying gratification. The required dosage is the sum of the estimated maintenance dose and a usual starting dose of an opioid. There is an incorrect patient belief or perception that methadone is not equi-analgesic to morphine (see Chapter 4). Methadone's NMDA antagonism property is indeed a theoretical

---

Box 12.1 Prerequisites for the use of opioids in terminally ill drug-abusing patients

1 Comprehensive clinical assessment: physical/psychosocial/psychiatric (including drug history)
2 Consent (informed, written)
3 Treatment agreement: prescribing 'rules', urine testing
4 Therapeutic analgesic trial
5 Collegial second opinion
6 Nominated single prescriber
7 Review, review, review (analgesia, aberrant behaviour, adverse reactions)

advantage. What remains pharmacologically mysterious is the required use of twice-daily dosing of methadone as an analgesic, but only once daily for drug dependency. Using a different opioid for analgesia in maintenance patients is favoured by some. Morphine and oxycodone may not be preferred because of their street appeal. The misuse potential of transdermal fentanyl is less, though straining fluid through the 'fentanyl tea-bag' is reported. Buprenorphine, which has mixed opioid agonism and antagonism (and can also be combined with low-dose naloxone), is another option.

It is difficult to ascertain the quantities of medicinal opioids diverted for illicit use. In India there were no reports of diversion from a home-based palliative care service,[10] whereas in the US misuse of oxycodone is 'widespread'.[11] While being cognisant of this risk, the prescriber's primary obligation is to the patient and the medicinally estimated requirement. Measures to try and reduce these risks are to provide supplies for short periods, random urine checks, not being accepting of the multiplicity of explanations and 'stories' about early exhaustion of supply, and eliciting family involvement in monitoring use (if in the home and the family are willing and capable). These patients are extraordinarily time consuming to manage. The most careful practitioner can be seduced by a clever and experienced drug seeker, who also has cancer. Possibly the most likely source of opioid drug diversion in palliative care is that of the 'wayward grandchild' who visits the dying grandparent with a purpose.

Anxiety disorders

Anxiety is an inevitable consequence of severe medical illness. In those predisposed to anxiety, the jags of enhanced anxieties during the course of illness are liable to exacerbate the underlying anxiety disorder. The anticipation of feared events can be worse than actually enduring of the event. Maintenance of existing anxiolytic regimes, both psychological and pharmacological, is critical. Boosting with additional therapies may be warranted. Preparatory information and reassurances concerning a necessary forthcoming procedure, the addition of short-term benzodiazepine, and the scheduling of extra psychotherapy sessions can be useful. Prophylactic anxiolysis with an SSRI (the most effective pharmacotherapeutic agent for persisting anxiety) warrants consideration. Those who appear psychologically fickle and vulnerable can surprise. Courage and fortitude are not related to anxiety.

Post-traumatic disorders

Those who have survived terrifying life-threatening experiences, events precipitating a chronic PTSD, may, when confronted with a terminal illness, experience a rekindling of the original trauma. The return of traumatic night terrors and intrusive thoughts, enhanced startle and flashbacks, all perhaps previously contained, again troubles the sick patient. This can be an early indicator of nervous system involvement of cancer. The cognitive impairment may result in the loss of the previously effective suppression and coping mechanisms. More probably, the illness serves to psychologically reactivate the veteran's past. This current confrontation with death reminds them of the previous occasions. Cachexia and weakness serve as physical cues to these memories.

PTSD has been conceptualised as an endogenous opioid deficiency state, similar to an opioid withdrawal syndrome.[12] Patients suffering PTSD have high substance use co-morbidity and propensity to self-medicate.[13,14] Opioid dysregulation occurs in PTSD.[15] The precise receptor involved is uncertain. Medicinal opioids and benzodiazepines serendipitously may relieve post-traumatic symptoms.

Intellectual disabilities

Emotions are often converted to behaviour in these patients. Grief may be expressed as bad, but really sad, behaviour. A change from usual behaviour should alert the carers to the possibility of a psychological cause. Insecure and over-protective developmental attachments are not uncommon.[16] Personality fragility compounds the intellectual limitations. Many intellectually disabled individuals are able to learn new information and from experience. But the learning is slow. When confronted with the crisis of serious illness the grasp of the information is laborious, if possible at all. Learning about aging, illness and death is delayed in those who are intellectually less able.[16] If living with family the mother–'child' bonding is likely to be intense, perhaps ambivalent. Communication may only be possible using the family as interpreters, who may not wish to relay the medical realities. While respecting the family's knowledge and intuitions, it is important to try to ascertain the patient's cognitive appraisal of their predicament.

References

1 Cervantes. *Don Quixote* (tr. JM Cohen). Harmondsworth: Penguin Books; 1952, pp. 936–8.

2 Macleod AD. Respiratory depression and melancholia. *Int J Psychiatry Med.* 1990; 20: 383–91.

3 Freud S. *Beyond the Pleasure Principle. The standard edition of the complete works, Vol XVII.* London: Hogarth Press; 1954, p. 33.

4 Borchardt CM and Popkin MK. Delirium and the resolution of depression. *J Clin Psychiatry.* 1987; 48: 373–5.

5 Talbot JA and Linn L. Reactions of schizophrenics to life-threatening disease. *Psychol Q.* 1987; 50: 218–27.

6 Goldenberg D, Holland J and Schachter S. Palliative care in the chronically mentally ill. In: Cochinov HM and Breitbart W (eds). *Handbook of Psychiatry in Palliative Medicine.* Oxford: Oxford University Press; 2000, pp. 91–6.

7 Browne T. *Christian Morals.* Pt.I, xxi. Quoted in *The Oxford Dictionary of Quotations: Third Edition.* London: Book Club Associates; 1981, p. 95.

8 Weissman DE and Haddox JD. Opioid pseudoaddiction – an iatrogenic syndrome. *Pain.* 1989; 36: 363–6.

9 Alford DP, Compton P and Samut JH. Acute pain management for patients receiving maintenance methadone or buprenorphine therapy. *Ann Intern Med.* 2006; 144: 127–34.

10 Rajagopal MR, Jorenson DE and Gilson AM. Medical use, abuse, and diversion of opioids in India. *Lancet.* 2001; 358: 118–23.

11 Cicero TJ, Inciardi JA and Munoz A. Trends in abuse of oxycontin and other opioids analgesics in the United States: 2002–2004. *J Pain*. 2005; 10: 662–72.

12 Kosten TR and Krystal J. biological mechanisms in PTSD: relevance for substance abuse. *Recent Dev Alcohol*. 1998; 6: 49–68.

13 Chilcoat HD and Breslau N. Post traumatic stress disorder and drug disorders: testing causal pathways. *Arch Gen Psychiatry*. 1998; 55: 913–17.

14 Bremner JD, Southwick SM, Darnell A, et al. Chronic PTSD in Vietnam combat veterans: course of illness and substance abuse. *Am J Psychiatry*. 1996; 153: 369–75.

15 Friedman MJ. What might the psychobiology of PTSD teach us about future approaches to pharmacotherapy? *J Clin Psychiatry*. 2000; 61(suppl 7): 44–51.

16 Blackman N. Supporting bereaved people with intellectual disabilities. *Eur J Palliat Care*. 2005; 12: 247–8.

Chapter 13

Euthanasia and psychiatry

Nor is death the worst we can look for; lingering life, and death denied, may be still deadlier.

Sophocles (496–406 BC)[1]

Historically medicine has been opposed to legalised euthanasia. The general public has a differing view and is increasingly vocal about the deficient care of the dying. Palliative medicine, psychiatry and general practice are starting to more studiously consider the complexities of these issues. Several specialist medical colleges in the UK have shifted to a neutral, rather than an opposed, stance. Legalised euthanasia and/or physician-assisted suicide (PAS) are practised in the Netherlands, Belgium, Estonia, Switzerland and the State of Oregon, USA. Valuable knowledge and opinion are being gained from these experiences. Euthanasia is a crisis that modern medicine must attend to. Psychiatry, unwillingly, has the key role in those jurisdictions in which euthanasia law has been passed, for it is the gatekeeper for euthanasia.

Whenever the Roman Emperor Augustus heard of anyone having passed away quickly and painlessly, he used to pray 'May Heaven grant the same euthanasia to me and mine'.[2] The quest for a good death, an easy death, painless and without suffering, remains elusive. The process of dying 'badly' (*eusthanasia* [f Gk hard, bad, unlucky death]) is an inherent fear, 'dying with dignity' a hope. Increasingly fear of dying rather than fear of death is a dominant concern of developed societies. An aging population and medical technology able to sustain life have influenced this changing anxiety. An 'appropriate death' has four

---

Box 13.1   Principles of a good death[3]

- To know when death is coming, and to understand what to expect
- To be able to retain control over what happens
- To be afforded dignity and privacy
- To have control over pain relief and other symptom control
- To have access to information and expertise of whatever kind necessary
- To have access to any spiritual and emotional support required
- To have access to hospice care in any location, not only hospital
- To have control over who is present and who shares the end
- To be able to issue advance directives which ensure wishes are respected
- To have time to say goodbye, and control over other aspects of timing
- To be able to leave when it is time to go, and not to have life prolonged pointlessly

---

outstanding characteristics: awareness, acceptance, propriety and timeliness.[4] Palliative medicine is committed to providing good symptom control and ultimately a good death (*see* Box 13.1).[3] The criteria for a 'good death' may be more easily fulfilled by euthanasia than by allowing nature autonomy. Public opinion polls suggest 80% support such legalisation in the UK.[5] Dutch studies have indicated that the closer the patient is to death the less common the requests. Compared to when initially diagnosed with cancer, only 26% were still considering euthanasia when death was imminent with advanced disease.[6] Proximity to death influences views. Requests for euthanasia are not uncommon in medical practice, though the literature is highly inaccurate. In a study published in 2000, up to 30% of Northern Ireland GPs over the preceding 5 years had been asked to perform euthanasia.[7] In North America 20% of physicians have received at least one request, 11% in Italy, and 45% in Australia.[8] In palliative medicine such requests are, however, rare occurrences.

Euthanasia is killing on request. PAS is defined as 'a doctor intentionally helping a person to commit suicide by providing drugs for self-administration, at the person's voluntary and competent request'.[9] Withholding futile treatment, withdrawing futile treatment, and terminal sedation are not considered euthanasia.[9]

The euthanasia debate

Over the last 50 years there has been a dramatic shift in both the location of death and the responsibility for the dying. Previously, families cared for their sick in the home and the care was governed by the personal, society and religious beliefs of these individuals. Now most deaths in developed countries occur in public institutions. The care is governed by the society mores. Issues about euthanasia have become common and public ones. Over the same period, medicine became scientifically capable of artificially sustaining life. For the first time the very sick have options of living or dying. Euthanasia debates do not occur in societies without health services sufficiently affluent to be able to keep persons artificially living.[10]

There are several core viewpoints presented within the debate:

1 *the right of autonomy*: individuals, particularly in Western countries, demand the right to choose if and when they die
2 *religious sanctions*: most traditional religions believe God decides time of death and not the individual
3 *suffering*: if severe and unrelieved then it is humane (with permission) to kill the sufferer
4 *financial*: the aging population will result in too few young persons able to care for their elderly, and investing funds to support and extend the nursing profession is not considered a priority. From a financial perspective, curtailing the duration of the final illness would be cost beneficial to a society
5 *the 'slippery slope'*: mankind is not responsible, as proven by history. The accepted criteria for euthanasia will eventually be exploited for political or other advantages.

The only one of these viewpoints of relevance to medicine (the profession rather than the individual) is that of suffering. Palliative care, the discipline, has, since its modern establishment, opposed legalised euthanasia. The viewpoint is that suffering can be relieved for the majority by palliative care expertise, and terminal sedation allows control of symptoms if all else proves ineffective.

Legalised physician-assisted suicide

In 1996, for the first time in history, a democratically elected government made both euthanasia and PAS legal. The following year the Australian government overturned this Northern Territory state law. In nine months, seven patients had made formal use of this law and four died under it.

In 1997 the State of Oregon, USA, legalised PAS, but not euthanasia. PAS accounted for only 0.1% of deaths in 2004.[11] The patient is prescribed a supply of lethal medication (a barbiturate) to be consumed orally. Between 1998 and 2004 only 326 prescriptions were given, and 208 ended their life this way (36% dying naturally).[11] The Oregon data suggest that patients do not request PAS because of unrelieved physical symptoms, or inadequacy of palliative care services (most are simultaneously enrolled in hospice programmes), and neither are they depressed or socially vulnerable.[12] They request assisted suicide for psychological and existential reasons: they value control, dread dependence on others, are ready to die, and assess current quality of life as poor.[12]

In the Netherlands, euthanasia and PAS have been sanctioned and practised openly since 1991. In 2001 PAS was made legal under certain circumstances and required to be reported to the coroner. About 5000 requests are made each year and this rate is now steady.[8] Cancer is the commonest diagnosis (74%, mainly gastrointestinal and lung), 7% have cardiovascular disease, and 5% severe pulmonary disease. The major reasons for the requests are fear of pain (37%), deteriorating physical status (31%), hopelessness (22%), and dyspnoea (15%). The diseases of those who made requests for PAS in 2000–2001 were physical disease (92.6%), psychiatric disease (2.9%) and 'weary of life' (4.5%).[13] The mean age of the requester was 67–68 years. Most were being nursed at home.[14] The most important concerns were non-physical.[14] Usually the concerns were multifactorial and included fears of dependence, loss of autonomy, loss of dignity, being a burden on others, and social isolation.[14] Loss of control appeared a core influencing factor. Of the three major factors the personal/social ones ('tired of life') were more relevant, encouraging the request, than the physical and psychiatric ones.[14] In the physical group, 42% of the requests were granted, none in the psychiatric group and 1% in the 'weary' group.[13] Suffering in the absence of severe disease is not an accepted indication for PAS.[13] The characteristics of the 400 'weary' patients were old age (average 81 years), 'reasonable' health, aloneness, and social isolation, but also 'through or tired of living and physically deteriorating'.[13] Only 50% of all euthanasia cases are estimated to be reported.[6] About 2.8% of all Dutch deaths are by euthanasia.[15] Belgium followed and legalised both PAS and euthanasia in 2002. Belgium is the only country where mental suffering from either somatic or mental disorder is explicitly acknowledged in law as a valid basis for euthanasia.[15] The mentally ill person must be competent, continuously suffering unbearably, and experiencing a severe and incurable disorder. To date most requests for those suffering mood disorders have been declined as there were still psychiatric treatment options left.[15] Euthanasia represents only 0.3% of all Belgian deaths. Termination of life on request (euthanasia) is more common in the Netherlands (2.4%), than Belgium (1.1%), while termination of life without request is more common in Belgium (3.2% versus 0.7%).[6]

Assisted suicide has been legally possible in Switzerland since 1937.[5]

Psychiatry in physician-assisted suicide jurisdictions

The objectives for psychiatric involvement in euthanasia requests, as detailed by legislators in the respective countries, are to determine mental competency and to evaluate mental ill-health. These are reasonable clinical tasks to be asked of psychiatry. However in the terminally ill these are not simple and straightforward clinical determinations.

In the Northern Territory, Australia the patient under the law had to be certified to be of sound mind and making the decision freely, voluntarily, and after due consideration.[15] A psychiatrist was required to examine the patient and confirm that the patient was not suffering from a 'treatable' clinical depression. Four of the seven patients considered (two died before the law came into effect, one after its repeal) had some symptoms of depression. One, despite current depressive symptoms and a probable subtherapeutic dose of antidepressant, was considered to be 'depressed consistent with her medical condition'. The other three to die were considered competent and not depressed. The psychiatric assessment was mandatory, raising concerns regarding co-operation, honesty and trust issues.[16] Indeed one patient assessed withheld relevant history.[16] No ongoing assessment or psychiatric treatment was offered or proposed. The psychiatrist merely functioned as the (open) gatekeeper to PAS in this situation. The opinions would appear to be at best cursory.

In the Netherlands physicians ask for a psychiatric evaluation for patients requesting PAS in only 3% of cases.[17] Since the law change in 2001 the person does not need to be competent when 'euthanased'. An advance request can be made, which remains valid despite altering health status. In 1995, of 4500 cases of active termination of life, 20% were without the patient's request.[6] Minors aged 16–18 years can request PAS, provided that the parents have been consulted (though they can not veto their adolescent's request). The Dutch medical fraternity believe that a person can have a death wish and not be clinically depressed.[13] How often requests are declined because of a co-existing depressive disorder is uncertain. Ultimately the decision to enact PAS rests on how the doctor considers the patient's suffering. It could be argued that it is not patients exerting autonomy, but doctors exercising power.[6] Objective criteria assessing suffering are neither available nor indeed possible. How the suffering is determined to be unbearable rests upon the impression of the assessing doctor.

In Oregon if the primary physician believes a psychiatric disorder is present, the patient must be referred to a psychiatrist or psychologist. The poor ability to detect psychiatric disorder by primary care physicians is well recognised.[17] Only 6% of psychiatrists were confident that on a single consultation they could determine if mental disorder was influencing the request. There is no established threshold for determining whether a patient is competent to choose suicide.[17] Depression (in Oregon) may or may not invalidate a voluntary request, and treatment of depression only improves the desire for life-sustaining therapy in a minority.[16–18]

The key task for psychiatry in Belgium is the assessment of competency in those whom the treating doctor thinks will not die in the foreseeable future.[15] These are generally those patients with mental illness. Competence is not defined in the law. Depressive disorder and demoralisation may influence the ability to rationally assimilate information and make decisions; psychiatric illnesses are not as well understood as diseases such as cancer and as yet there is considerable uncertainty (and criticism) about the practice of this aspect of the Belgian law.[15]

The current provision of psychiatric assessment, as legislated in these jurisdictions, would appear to be inadequate to perform the task expected. The current knowledge of the psychiatry of the terminally ill, and experience to date in these countries, raises the probability that the legal expectation of psychiatry is not achievable.

The problems for psychiatry

Individualism versus professionalism

The psychological issues of the doctor are relevant. The fatigued, hopeless and despairing doctor confronted by a patient requesting assisted suicide may more easily acquiesce or subtly encourage the act.[19] The psychiatrist's personal values and beliefs about PAS may be more influential than professional knowledge upon determination.[20] The professional views of the doctor about PAS are highly correlated with their personal views of this practice.[21] Making the ultimate decision regarding the ability to bear suffering, as the doctor is expected to in the Netherlands, is likely more influenced by individual than professional views.

Hippocratic medicine professes to do no harm. Killing patients is a role doctors neither wish nor want. Anaesthetists, potential executioners because of their skills inducing states of unresponsiveness, are firmly opposed.[22] Indirect killing as in Oregon, or by a state-appointed executioner, are obvious options, but hardly fulfil the medical obligation of non-abandonment (*see* Chapter 3).

Assessing competency

The prevalence of psychological distress and psychiatric illness in the dying is high. Affectations of the brain and mind influence judgement and decision making. Determining mental fitness to decide upon life-sustaining or relieving options is at best imprecise (*see* Chapter 10). Assessing competency is difficult, as the capabilities required to decide on suicide are not known. That 20% non-competent persons die by PAS in the Netherlands certainly provokes concern of a 'slippery slope'.

Depression and the desire for death

The effect mood and anxiety have upon cognitive functioning and decision making is very relevant (*see* Chapters 2 and 6).

In persons over the age of 65 years, 9.5% have suicidal thoughts, but only 0.14% actually attempt suicide.[23] High desire to die is present in 5–10% of the palliative care population. Persistent requests for euthanasia are uncommon in palliative care practice, though more frequent in primary care. In severely ill patients, the will to live fluctuates.[24] The will to live is determined more strongly by psychological variables until the last few days when supplanted by physical variables such as pain and dyspnoea.[25] In terminally ill cancer patients, psychological distress rather than pain and functional status is the most influential factor determining the desire to die.[24] The strongest factors are hopelessness, depression and anxiety.[26] Major depression was diagnosed in 59% of hospice patients who persistently desired a hastened death, but in only 8% of those who did not.[24] The wish to die is not stable, especially if mental health problems are evident.[27] Those who received substantive intervention such as control of pain, hospice referral, psychosocial and antidepressant medication, were more likely to change their mind about PAS.[27] They also had less advanced disease. Only 11% changed their mind after an antidepressant trial.[27] Those whose decision altered were more ambivalent and unstable with regard to the initial request, not as hopeless, and had a few treatment options still available.[8] In the Netherlands 13% had a change of mind. This was less likely in the terminal phase and more likely if there were mental health problems.[8] Instability of attitude concerning PAS, generally toward rejection of an earlier supportive view, occurred in 8–26%, particularly if depression lifted.[28] In Oregon, no PAS patient has contacted emergency services after consuming the lethal medication, though this would need to be done within 25 minutes.[11]

Fluctuating will to live and desire to die occur in a significant proportion of terminally ill. If clinically depressed, the desire to die is more likely, though with intervention change is infrequent. Existential variables have a stronger effect on the desire to die than psychological and psychiatric ones.[29] Desire for death may be driven by the intolerable future rather than the intolerable present.[30] Spiritual wellbeing (a sense of meaning and peace) is an important modifier of the desire to die, and even if depressed, it is protective.[31] The percentages of patients changing their view about PAS, perhaps 10–15%, while small, would be considered to be an unacceptably high operating mortality in surgical practice. Of additional concern, and possibly influential in oncological practice, is the impression that by offering further treatment options, a view about euthanasia may alter.[8] However these patients had lesser disease burden and this may be of greater relevance.

Fears of dying

> When hope goes, uncertainty goes too, and men don't fear uncertainty.
> Admiral Richard Byrd (1938)[32]

The fear of dying is universal (*see* Chapter 2). Often this concerns the process more than the event. Uncertainty incites anxiety. Dying patients are more anxious if death seems probable rather than certain.[33] Admiral Byrd, trapped in the Antarctic winter, alone and unable to be rescued, experienced that having accepted the inevitability of his death, his anxiousness settled.[32] Knowing a date of death may flood and then diminish anxieties and fears. Socrates was free of dread before he drank the hemlock, saying 'that to be afraid of death is only another form of thinking that one is wise when one is not; it is to think one knows what one does not know'.[34] The inherent fears of dying and death are amplified by the enhancing public perception that modern medicine will resuscitate and sustain life even in those with little prospect of good quality of life. Advance directives are driven, albeit slowly, by such concerns. Ongoing public relations exercises by medical researchers that they are on the verge of solving a disease perpetuate these beliefs. Euthanasia is a reaction to the fear of being 'kept alive when dead'.

The process of dying is becoming increasingly fraught and difficult. This is a cost of the curing philosophy of modern medicine. Assertive oncological treatments, aimed only to prolong life for weeks to months, are allowing cancer patients to live longer. This also allows the accumulation of disease in multiple organs, including the brain. Ultimately the terminal phase of life is influenced by multiple partial organ dysfunctions and failures. It is probable because of this that the prevalence of terminal delirium is increasing. The acute mortality of cancer has been arrested. Cancer has been converted into a chronic illness with a more complicated death. Many are treated assertively up to and including the dying stage. Medicine has seemingly lost its clinical judgement and wisdom. It is easier to do what is technically possible to be done than to consider wisely the quality of life. Johann Stieglitz (1767–1840) stated 'I have often thought it would be important to instruct physicians how to behave in cases of incurable disease: not so much to tell them what to do; rather what not to do'.[35] In the 21st century this thought is even more pertinent. There was always for Hippocrates a fundamental question: to treat or not to treat? Making prognoses was a primary medical function. To help, or at least do no harm, was the Hippocratic tradition. Modern medicine is predominantly taught in large technologically sophisticated hospitals by medical researchers with interests in curing rather than caring. Doctors are not trained to be sensible and sensitive clinicians. Expert clinicians have been devalued in recent decades within medicine. Making a good bedside diagnosis of dying, and addressing the situation rather than enacting a procedure, is a skill some learn by experience, but many never learn. That modern medicine's care of the dying is deficient ignites in the general public the simplistic response that orchestrating euthanasia would be a solution.

The time of death

All dais (days) march toward death, only the last comes to it.
Michel de Montaigne (1533–1592)[36]

Making accurate prognoses about the time of death is medically difficult. Not only are there rafts of physiological variables, there are also psychological ones. All those who work in palliative care recognise that individuals can postpone death a short while to participate in an important event, and alternatively 'will' death if ready. The Sabbath effect, the reduced probability of death on the Sabbath, has been shown in an Israeli population,[37] though a large US population study of deaths at Christmas, Thanksgiving and birthdays did not suggest that cancer patients could postpone death.[38] The involvement of the nervous system, which needs to be considered in investigating this issue, would probably negate any psychological effect on the timing of death. It is unlikely that the skill and knowledge to accurately determine time of death will easily be acquired, particularly as the natural history of cancers is so influenced by medical interventions, and investigating predilections (or otherwise) of death is difficult. Sanitising death is unnatural and may be disturbing for relatives, though so may be waiting, particularly if this period is agonising for patient and family. PAS has been shown to cause fewer traumatic grief symptoms in the bereaved family.[39] Hospice workers are familiar with the rich and rewarding time many families endure but appreciate during the vigil awaiting the death of a loved one. Oregon has shown that it is a myth that excellent palliative care is incompatible with legal access to PAS.[30] Good palliative care improves the outcome of grief for the relatives, but as yet it is uncertain how important being able to anticipate the timing of death might be.

Suicide versus physician-assisted suicide

Suicide is the voluntary and intentional taking of one's own life. Suicide is relatively infrequent in cancer patients (*see* Chapter 6). 'Psychological autopsy' studies suggest that 80% of persons with cancer who committed suicide were clinically depressed, about the same as for those suicides without cancer.[40] Suicide prevention has become a major public health issue in response to growing prevalence in groups of the community, particularly youth. Practising PAS appears inconsistent with these directives, and provides the general public a contradictory message. Finlay raises the relevant clinical observation that terminally ill patients are reluctant to kill themselves, yet some wish to be killed by their doctor.[41] Suicide and PAS are perceived to be different by the terminally ill.

Euthanasia and medicine

Relatively rarely do patients present to palliative care requesting euthanasia. If they do, the clinical problems initiating the request (in developed countries) are psychosocial and existential rather than medical or psychiatric. Doctors working in the community are more likely to field a request for euthanasia. The experience in the Netherlands suggests that some of these persons have no severe illness. Perhaps in other countries medical services are entirely unaware of this group of sufferers. Neither is it known if the existential factors initiating the request are in any way remediable to intervention.

There are many concerns regarding the oscillations of the will to die, the effect of depression on euthanasia requests, and what constitutes fitness to commit rational suicide. Psychology and psychiatry's challenge is to better understand these influences so they can perform credibly as gatekeepers, if legally requested to do so. Concerns of a 'slippery slope' remain. Subjective impression of suffering needs to be supplanted by solid objective evidence-based literature and clinical guidelines. Medicine has a responsibility to relearn to care for individual sick persons, to teach these skills and to temper curative hopes and aspirations. Dying needs to be better managed.

Every medical clinician in palliative medicine has attended individuals whose state of unremitting suffering appears unbearable, and whose wish for euthanasia is persistent. Terminal sedation is an effective and fair option for these patients.

It is not euthanasia by another name, and is an effective and appreciated medical intervention. Medicine can only opine on the association of suffering and euthanasia. Mostly this suffering has little or no disease involvement. Other than advocating caution for the above reasons, medicine has little to contribute. Attending better to the clinical process of dying would decrease euthanasia requests. The euthanasia issue will not vanish from modern society. Medicine and psychiatry need to start contributing to the debate rather than merely dismissing euthanasia as wrong.

References

1   Sophocles. Electra. *Electra and other plays* (tr. EF Watling). Harmondsworth: Penguin Books; 1953, p. 98.
2   Suetonius. Augustus. *The Twelve Caesars* (tr. R Graves). Harmondsworth: Penguin; 1957, p. 106.
3   Smith R. 'A good death' (editorial). *BMJ.* 2000; 320: 129–30.
4   Weisman AD. *The Vulnerable Self: confronting the ultimate questions.* New York: Insight Books, Plenum Press; 1993, pp. 190–6.
5   Branthwaite MA. Time for change. *BMJ.* 2005; 331: 681–3.
6   ten Have H. Why not legalise euthanasia and physician-assisted suicide? *Eur J Palliat Care.* 2003; 10(suppl): 21–7.
7   McGlade KJ, Slaney L, Bunting BP *et al.* Voluntary euthanasia in Northern Ireland: general practitioner's beliefs, experiences, and actions. *Br J Gen Pract.* 2000; 50: 794–7.
8   Marcoux I, Onwuteaka-Philipsen BD, Jansen-van der Weide MC *et al.* Withdrawing an explicit request for euthanasia or physician-assisted suicide: a retrospective study on the influence of mental health status and other patient characteristics. *Psychol Med.* 2005; 35: 1265–74.
9   Materstvedt LJ, Clark D, Ellershaw J *et al.* Euthanasia and physician-assisted suicide: a view from an EAPC Ethics Task Force. *Palliat Med.* 2003; 17: 97–101.
10 Spence D. From the West Indies. *Palliat Med.* 2003; 17: 155.
11 Okie S. Physician-assisted suicide: Oregon and beyond. *N Eng J Med.* 2005; 352: 1627–30.
12 Ganzini L and Back A. From the USA: understanding requests for physician-assisted death. *Palliat Med.* 2003; 17: 113–14.
13 Rurup ML, Muller MT, Onwuteaka-Philipsen BD *et al.* Requests for euthanasia or physician-assisted suicide from older persons who do not have a severe disease: an interview study. *Psychol Med.* 2005; 35: 665–71.
14 Marquet RL, Bartelds A, Visser GJ *et al.* Twenty five years of requests for euthanasia and physician assisted euthanasia in Dutch general practice: trend analysis. *BMJ.* 2003; 327: 201–2.
15 Naudts K, Ducatelle C, Kovacs J *et al.* Euthanasia: the role of the psychiatrist. *Br J Psychiatry.* 2006; 188: 405–9.
16 Kissane DK, Street A and Nitschke P. Seven deaths in Darwin: case studies under the Rights of the Terminally Ill Act, Northern Territory, Australia. *Lancet.* 1998; 352: 1097–102.
17 Ganzini L and Lee MA. Psychiatry and assisted suicide in the United States (editorial). *N Eng J Med.* 1997; 336: 1824–6.
18 Ganzini L, Lee MA, Heintz RT *et al.* The effect of depression treatment on elderly patient's preferences for life-sustaining medical treatment. *Am J Psychiatry.* 1994; 151: 1631–6.
19 Miles S. Physicians and their patient's suicides. *JAMA.* 1994; 271: 1786–8.

20 Zauber TS and Sullivan MD. Psychiatry and physician-assisted suicide. *Psychiatr Clin North Am.* 1996; 19: 413–27.

21 Ganzini L, Fenn DS, Lee MA *et al.* Attitudes of Oregon psychiatrists toward physician-assisted suicide. *Am J Psychiatry.* 1996; 153: 1469–75.

22 Jonsen AR. To help the dying die – a new duty for anesthesiologists? (editorial). *Anesthesiology.* 1993; 78: 225–8.

23 Scocco P and De Leo D. One-year prevalence of death thoughts, suicide ideation and behaviours in an elderly population. *Int J Geriatr Psychiatry.* 2002; 17: 842–6.

24 Cochinov HM, Wilson KG, Enns M *et al.* Desire for death in the terminally ill. *Am J Psychiatry.* 1995; 152: 1185–91.

25 Cochinov HM, Tataryn D, Clinch JJ *et al.* Will to live in the terminally ill. *Lancet.* 1999; 354: 816–19.

26 Mystakidou K, Rosenfeld B, Parpa E *et al.* Desire for death near the end of life: the role of depression, anxiety and pain. *Gen Hosp Psychiatry.* 2005; 27: 258–62.

27 Ganzini L, Nelson HD, Schmidt TA *et al.* Physician's experiences with the Oregon Death with Dignity Act. *N Eng J Med.* 2000; 342: 557–63.

28 Blank K, Robison J, Prigerson H *et al.* Instability of attitudes about euthanasia and physician assisted euthanasia in depressed older hospitalised patients. *Gen Hosp Psychiatry.* 2001; 23: 326–32.

29 Cochinov HM, Hack T, Hassard T *et al.* Understanding the will to live in patients nearing death. *Psychosomatics.* 2005; 46: 7–10.

30 Sullivan MD. The desire for death arises from an intolerable future rather than an intolerable present. *Gen Hosp Psychiatry.* 2005; 27: 256–7.

31 McClain-Jacobson C, Rosenfeld B, Kosinski A *et al.* Belief in an afterlife, spiritual well-being in patients with advanced cancer. *Gen Hosp Psychiatry.* 2004; 26: 484–6.

32 Byrd RE. *Alone: the classic polar adventure.* New York: Kondansha America, Inc; 1995, p.181 (original publication. New York: Putnam's Sons; 1938).

33 Hinton J. The progress of awareness and acceptance of dying assessed in cancer patients and their caring relatives. *Palliat Med.* 1999; 13: 19–35.

34 Plato. *The Last Days of Socrates: The Apology of Socrates.* (tr. H Tredennick) Harmondsworth: Penguin Books; 1954, p. 34.

35 Stieglitz J. Letter to Dr Karl FH Marx, December 15, 1826. Quoted in MB Strauss (ed). *Familiar Medical Quotations.* Boston: Little, Brown and Company; 1968, p. 237.

36 Montaigne M. That to Philosophie Is to Learn to Die. *The Essays of Montaigne done into English by John Florio.* Bk. I, Ch. 19. New York: AMS Press; 1967, p. 89.

37 Anson J and Anson O. Death rests a while: holy day and Sabbath effects on Jewish mortality in Israel. *Soc Sci Med.* 2001; 52: 83–97.

38 Young DC and Hade EM. Holidays, birthdays, and postponement of cancer death. *JAMA.* 2004; 292: 3012–16.

39 Swarte NB, van der Lee ML, van der Bom JG *et al.* Effects of euthanasia on the bereaved family and friends: a cross sectional study. *BMJ.* 327: 189–92.

40 Henrikson MM, Isometsa ET, Hietanen PS *et al.* Mental disorders in cancer suicides. *J Affect Disord.* 1995; 36: 11–20.

41 Finlay I. From the UK. *Palliat Med.* 2003; 17: 137.

Chapter 14

Psychopharmacology

> In all things there is a poison, and there is nothing without a poison. It depends only upon the dose whether a poison is poison or not.
>
> Paracelsus (1493–1541)[1]

Pharmacokinetics in the dying

The absorption, distribution, metabolism and excretion of drugs are affected by genetic and disease factors. Gut transit times, route of administration, loss of body mass, low albumin, dehydration, renal and hepatic failure may all influence pharmacokinetics. Smoking can reduce the blood concentrations of some psychotropic medications by as much as 50%, by the induction of cytochrome P450 (CYP) enzymes leading to an increase in metabolism. Grapefruit juice can enhance the concentrations of oral benzodiazepines. Drug interactions also affect drug concentrations. 'Start low, go slow' and the reduction of drug dosages in terminal illnesses are pharmacologically sensible clinical guidelines.

Placebo responses

Placebo effects in clinical trials are typically substantial and often account for the larger proportion of the improvement attributed to the therapeutic agent being tested. Pain and mood are particularly sensitive to a placebo impact. Expectation of effect, conditioning and learning are relevant mechanisms implying that both conscious and unconscious factors operate.[2] The benefit of extra attention afforded subjects participating in drug trials may result in more significant placebo effects than in usual clinical practice. Biological (e.g. sympathetic nervous system) as well as psychological parameters can be altered by a placebo. Functional imaging suggests involvement of prefrontal cortex and thalamic structures in the placebo effect. Serotonin has been implicated.[3] Hidden or secretive placebo administration is less effective than openly providing a 'dummy medication'.[2] The ethics of concealing a treatment preclude such a method.

Ethnic and cultural factors

Individual and inter-ethnic differences in the metabolism of some medications are substantial.[4,5] The rate-limiting steps in the metabolism of most psychotropic drugs are the CYP enzymes.[4] Ethnic variation exists in the CYP enzyme system. Genetic variations mainly determine the activity of these enzymes. Asian patients are more likely to experience extrapyramidal side-effects of antipsychotic

161

medications, and at lower dosage than Caucasian patients.[4] Asian and Hispanic patients metabolise tricyclic antidepressants more slowly, thus may require lower doses. This may also apply to benzodiazepines. Treatment adherence may be influenced by many factors including culture, medical belief systems, and linguistic misunderstandings.

References

1 Jacobi J. *Paracelsus: Selected Writings*. Princeton: Princeton University Press; 1998, p. 95.
2 Benedetti F. Recent advances in placebo research. *Int J Pain Med Palliat Care*. 2005; 4: 2–7.
3 Mayberg H, Silva JA, Brannan SK *et al*. The functional neuroanatomy of the placebo effect. *Am J Psychiatry*. 2002; 159: 728–37.
4 Lim K-M, Smith M and Ortiz V. Culture and psychopharmacology. *Psychiatr Clin N Am*. 2001; 24: 523–38.
5 Bhugra D and Bhui K. Ethnic and cultural factors in psychopharmacology. *Adv Psychiatric Treat*. 1999; 5: 89–95.

Index